Decision Making for Minimally Invasive Spine Surgery

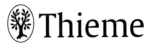

Decision Making for Minimally Invasive Spine Surgery

Faheem A. Sandhu, MD, PhD
Associate Professor
Director of Spine Surgery
Department of Neurosurgery
Georgetown University Hospital
Washington, DC

Jean-Marc Voyadzis, MD
Assistant Professor
Department of Neurosurgery
Georgetown University Hospital
Washington, DC

Richard G. Fessler, MD, PhD
Professor
Department of Neurosurgery
Northwestern University Feinberg School of Medicine
Chicago, Illinois

Thieme
New York • Stuttgart

Thieme Medical Publishers, Inc.
333 Seventh Ave.
New York, NY 10001

Executive Editor: Kay Conerly
Managing Editor: Dominik Pucek
Editorial Director, Clinical Reference: Michael Wachinger
Production Editor: Kenny Chumbley, Publication Services
International Production Director: Andreas Schabert
Vice President, International Marketing and Sales: Cornelia Schulze
Chief Financial Officer: James W. Mitos
President: Brian D. Scanlan
Compositor: Publication Services
Printer: Transcontinental Printing

Library of Congress Cataloging-in-Publication Data

Decision making for minimally invasive spine surgery / [edited by] Faheem A. Sandhu, Jean-Marc Voyadzis, Richard G. Fessler.
  p. ; cm.
  Includes bibliographical references and index.
  Summary: "The art and science of spinal surgery has been in constant evolution since the early middle ages. The majority of advances, however, have occurred after World War II with the advent of antibiotics, better imaging, improved diagnostic methods, and surgical care. In the past five to ten years, a greater understanding of spinal anatomy and the development of more sophisticated radiological imaging and instrumentation have further illuminated what is possible in spinal care. Decision Making for Minimally Invasive Spine Surgery adds to the historical continuum by compiling a collection of chapters that define why a minimally invasive approach should be chosen and how to perform such a procedure, written by authors who have established themselves as experts in the field"—Provided by publisher.
  ISBN 978-1-60406-266-3 (alk. paper)
  1. Spine—Surgery. 2. Spine—Endoscopic surgery. 3. Decision making. I. Sandhu, Faheem A. II. Voyadzis, Jean-Marc. III. Fessler, Richard G.
  [DNLM: 1. Spinal Diseases—surgery. 2. Decision Making. 3. Spine—surgery. 4. Surgical Procedures, Minimally Invasive—methods. WE 725]
  RD768.D42   2011
  617.5'6059—dc22
                                                                    2010041698

Important note: Medical knowledge is ever-changing. As new research and clinical experience broaden our knowledge, changes in treatment and drug therapy may be required. The authors and editors of the material herein have consulted sources believed to be reliable in their efforts to provide information that is complete and in accord with the standards accepted at the time of publication. However, in view of the possibility of human error by the authors, editors, or publisher of the work herein or changes in medical knowledge, neither the authors, editors, nor publisher, nor any other party who has been involved in the preparation of this work, warrants that the information contained herein is in every respect accurate or complete, and they are not responsible for any errors or omissions or for the results obtained from use of such information. Readers are encouraged to confirm the information contained herein with other sources. For example, readers are advised to check the product information sheet included in the package of each drug they plan to administer to be certain that the information contained in this publication is accurate and that changes have not been made in the recommended dose or in the contraindications for administration. This recommendation is of particular importance in connection with new or infrequently used drugs.

Some of the product names, patents, and registered designs referred to in this book are in fact registered trademarks or proprietary names even though specific reference to this fact is not always made in the text. Therefore, the appearance of a name without designation as proprietary is not to be construed as a representation by the publisher that it is in the public domain.

Printed in Canada

978-1-60406-266-3

To Henna, Zain, Rafae, Sabrina, and my parents for love, patience, and guidance.

Faheem A. Sandhu

To my parents, Spiros and Claudine, and my sister, Sandra, for their love and unwavering support.

Jean-Marc Voyadzis

To my wife, Carol, whose dedication to my health and well being, our family, and to my career not only ensured success in each of those areas, but whose presence made each day a gift to be anticipated. For all you have sacrificed over the years, thank you.

Richard G. Fessler

Contents

Foreword

The art and science of spinal surgery has been in constant evolution since the early middle ages. The majority of advances, however, have occurred after World War II with the advent of antibiotics, better imaging, improved diagnostic methods, and surgical care. In the past five to ten years, a greater understanding of spinal anatomy and the development of more sophisticated radiological imaging and instrumentation have further illuminated what is possible in spinal care. *Decision Making for Minimally Invasive Spine Surgery* adds to the historical continuum by compiling a collection of chapters that define why a minimally invasive approach should be chosen and how to perform such a procedure, written by authors who have established themselves as experts in the field.

Minimally invasive techniques may not be for every surgeon, but more likely than not, some aspects of minimally invasive surgery will appeal to the modern spine surgeon, even those with particular expertise in the correction of spinal deformities. Unfortunately, the current learning curve for minimally invasive procedures is longer than in traditional surgery, and it is still somewhat uncertain whether the investment will net a provable return. For example, the complications of mini-open fusion versus traditional open surgery are the same in an overall literature search, though the fusion rates are slightly less for the former. The length of hospital stay and return to work (activities) has certainly decreased compared to conventional methods but at some risk of increased radiation exposure. Finally, are the savings sufficient to overcome the possible increased complication rate for minimally invasive procedures? Which option is the right one, and for which case?

The authors have attempted to answer these questions and in my opinion have succeeded. This book is unique in that the authors present an authoritative text with a focus on evaluative questions to make a strong determination as to which approach would be best for the patient. To that end, algorithms have been designed for the specific pathology that is addressed at the start of each chapter to assist the reader in the selection of minimally invasive treatment over traditional open surgery. The book closes with a look at image guidance and instrumentation systems, as well as a discussion of what the coming state of the art will be. Experienced neurosurgeons, orthopedic surgeons, and spine surgeons will find this book a useful resource when considering the option of minimally invasive surgery, whereas residents and spine fellows who have a growing interest in the specialty will look to this as an invaluable guide in acquiring and refining new skills.

Having been known as a maximally invasive surgeon, particularly as the surgery applies to deformity, I am firmly convinced that minimally invasive spinal surgery is here to stay and will advance. This text goes a long way in supporting this thesis.

John P. Kostuik, MD
Professor Emeritus
Orthopaedics/Neurosurgery
Johns Hopkins University
Baltimore, Maryland
Chairman and Chief Medical Officer
K2M Incorporated
Leesburg, Virginia

Preface

For many years the desire for less invasive procedures has been forged by patients and surgeons alike. A wealth of recent technological advances in the field of spinal surgery has made it possible to satisfy this desire. The development of unique retractor systems, along with the refinement of osteobiologics, and advances in endoscopy, fluoroscopy, and frameless navigation have allowed spinal surgeons to treat the breadth of spinal disease with less invasive means, from diskectomy and decompression, to arthrodesis and even spinal deformity. An exponentially growing number of publications demonstrate the safety and efficacy of these techniques, in essence proving the assertion that these procedures *can* be done and to great benefit. Nonetheless, the obvious advantages of limited tissue dissection, decreased blood loss, and faster recovery are often tempered with a lack of clinical superiority when compared with conventional techniques, leaving surgeons to wonder if it is really worthwhile to learn new, possibly more difficult and time consuming procedures when their current practice yields excellent results. Minimally invasive techniques offer distinct advantages in certain clinical settings and *should* be considered the preferred treatment method for some, but certainly not all spinal conditions. That said, determining when or why a less invasive technique should be adopted is difficult to ascertain from attending meetings, taking courses, or by reading journals alone.

The principal goal of this book is to provide a comprehensive look at the current advantages and limitations of minimally invasive spinal procedures (MIS) as compared with conventional methods to guide both novice and experienced spine surgeons in deciding on the optimal treatment strategy for a given spinal problem. Our intent is to remove some of the sensationalism that surrounds minimally invasive spine surgery and to provide a concrete rationale for choosing a less invasive approach over a conventional one, and vice versa. For example, in the average patient, the effectiveness of minimally invasive lumbar diskectomy performed with tubular retractors is equivalent to standard open microdiscectomy. However, the use of tubular retractors is far more advantageous in the morbidly obese patient, which is also true for far lateral lumbar diskectomy. In an effort to encourage spine surgeons to invest in acquiring and performing minimally invasive techniques, we have provided a flowchart at the beginning of each chapter to summarize and aid the decision-making process for various approaches and conditions of the cervical, thoracic, and lumbar spine.

Preserving as much of the normal anatomic structure of the spine while simultaneously addressing the underlying pathology is the essence of minimally invasive spinal surgery. The ability to minimize the disruption of surrounding spinal elements has evolved to more than simply the use of tubular retractors and endoscopes. Choosing the right approach under the appropriate circumstances and performing it safely in a time and cost effective manner will be the measure of success for MIS procedures in the long term. We hope that this book provides insight into this complex decision-making process and promotes the use of minimally invasive techniques where and when it has the potential to yield the greatest outcome.

Faheem A. Sandhu
Jean-Marc Voyadzis
Richard G. Fessler

Acknowledgments

We would like to recognize all spine surgeons who have had the patience and courage to innovate and implement in an effort to improve patient care.

Contributors

Frank L. Acosta Jr., MD
Director of Spine Deformity
Department of Neurosurgery
Cedars-Sinai Medical Center
Los Angeles, California

Amjad N. Anaizi, MD
Resident
Department of Neurosurgery
Georgetown University Hospital
Washington, DC

Etevaldo Coutinho, MD
Instituto de Patologia da Coluna
Sao Paulo, Brazil

Richard G. Fessler, MD, PhD
Professor
Department of Neurosurgery
Northwestern University Feinberg
  School of Medicine
Chicago, Illinois

Vishal C. Gala, MD, MPH
Atlanta Brain and Spine Care
Atlanta, Georgia

Peter C. Gerszten, MD, MPH, FACS
Associate Professor
Department of Neurological Surgery
  and Radiation Oncology
University of Pittsburgh Medical Center
Pittsburgh, Pennsylvania

Regis W. Haid Jr., MD
Medical Director
Piedmont Spine Center
Piedmont Hospital
Director
Neuroscience Service Line
Piedmont Healthcare System
Atlanta, Georgia

Robert E. Isaacs, MD
Director of Spine Surgery
Division of Neurosurgery
Duke University School of Medicine
Durham, North Carolina

Isaac O. Karikari, MD
Resident
Division of Neurosurgery
Duke University School of Medicine
Durham, North Carolina

Larry T. Khoo, MD
Director of Neurological and Spine
  Surgery
The Spine Clinic of Los Angeles
Los Angeles, California

John C. Liu, MD
Associate Professor of Neurosurgery
Department of Neurosurgery
Northwestern University Feinberg
  School of Medicine
Chicago, Illinois

David J. Moller, MD
Assistant Professor
Department of Neurological Surgery
University of California–Davis
Davis, California

Edward A. Monaco III, MD, PhD
Resident
Department of Neurological Surgery
University of Pittsburgh Medical Center
Pittsburgh, Pennsylvania

Pierce D. Nunley, MD
Clinical Associate Professor
Chief of Spine Service
Department of Orthopaedic Surgery
Louisiana State University Health
  Sciences Center
Shreveport, Louisiana

Eric K. Oermann, BS
Department of Neurosurgery
Georgetown University Hospital
Washington, DC

Leonardo Oliveira, MD
Instituto de Patologia da Coluna
Sao Paulo, Brazil

John O'Toole, MD
Assistant Professor
Department of Neurosurgery
Rush University Medical Center
Chicago, Illinois

Luiz H. M. Pimenta, MD, PhD
Associate Professor
University of California–San Diego
San Diego, California
Founder and Director
Instituto de Patologia Coluna
Sao Paulo, Brazil

Eric A. Potts, MD
Assistant Professor
Department of Neurological Surgery
Indiana University School of Medicine
Goodman Campbell Brain and Spine
Indianapolis, Indiana

Faheem A. Sandhu, MD, PhD
Associate Professor
Director of Spine Surgery
Department of Neurosurgery
Georgetown University Hospital
Washington, DC

Amanda Muhs Saratsis, MD
Resident
Department of Neurosurgery
Georgetown University Hospital
Washington, DC

Zachary A. Smith, MD
Fellow in Spine Surgery
The Spine Clinic of Los Angeles
Los Angeles, California

Sathish J. Subbaiah, MD
Assistant Professor
Department of Neurosurgery
Mount Sinai School of Medicine
New York, New York

Rikin A. Trivedi, MRCP (UK),
 FRCS(SN), PhD
Consultant Neurosurgeon
Addenbrooke's Hospital
Cambridge, United Kingdom

Jean-Marc Voyadzis, MD
Assistant Professor
Department of Neurosurgery
Georgetown University Hospital
Washington, DC

Michael Y. Wang, MD, FACS
Associate Professor
Departments of Neurological Surgery
  and Rehabilitation Medicine
University of Miami Miller School of
  Medicine
Miami, Florida

Section I

Cervical Spine

A

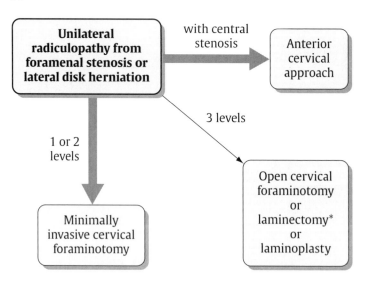

B

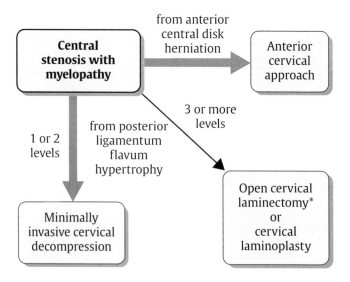

* With fusion if cervical kyphosis present.

1

Posterior Minimally Invasive Cervical Foraminotomy and Laminectomy

John O'Toole, Jean-Marc Voyadzis, and Vishal C. Gala

Posterior decompressive procedures are an essential component of the spinal surgeon's armamentarium in the surgical treatment of symptomatic cervical degenerative spine disease.[1-4] Although in recent years anterior cervical procedures have gained prominence, posterior cervical laminoforaminotomy remains of proven benefit, providing symptomatic relief in 92 to 97% of patients with radiculopathy from foraminal stenosis or lateral herniated disks.[3,5] Similarly, posterior cervical decompression for cervical stenosis results in neurological improvement in 62.5 to 83% of myelopathic patients undergoing either laminectomy or laminoplasty.[4,6-8] Moreover, these operations avoid the complications attendant on anterior approaches to the cervical spine, in particular, esophageal injury, vascular injury, recurrent laryngeal nerve paralysis, dysphagia, and accelerated degeneration of adjacent motion segments after fusion, or so-called adjacent segment disease.[9-11]

Open posterior approaches to the cervical spine require extensive subperiosteal stripping of the paraspinal musculature that often results in significant postoperative pain, muscle spasm, and dysfunction that can be permanently disabling in 18 to 60% of patients.[4,9,12,13] Furthermore, long-segment decompression in the patient who has a preoperative loss of lordosis increases the risk for postoperative sagittal plane deformity[14-17] and is typically an indication for instrumented arthrodesis at the time of laminectomy. Application of standard, extensive posterior fusion techniques increases operative time, surgical risks, and blood loss; exacerbates early postoperative pain; and potentially contributes to adjacent segment disease.

The fundamental tenet of minimal access techniques is the reduction of approach-related morbidity. To that end, the advent of muscle-splitting tubular retractor systems and their accompanying instruments, together with improvements in endoscopic technology, has allowed for the application of minimally invasive techniques to posterior cervical decompressive procedures.[13,18] Cervical microendoscopic foraminotomy/diskectomy (CMEF/D) was first described in a cadaver model and subsequently was shown to have clinical efficacy equivalent to that of traditional open procedures.

Cervical microendoscopic decompression of stenosis (CMEDS) is based upon more familiar techniques that have already been applied to cases of lumbar stenosis.[19] By preserving much of the normal osteoligamentous anatomy of the cervical spine, the CMEDS procedure reduces the risk of postlaminectomy kyphosis as well as difficulties associated with postlaminectomy membrane formation.[4,16]

◆ Preoperative Evaluation

Unilateral radicular symptoms that correlate with radiographic and electrophysiologic findings are ideally suited for CMEF/D, depending upon the underlying pathology. **Figure 1.1A** shows a soft lateralized disk herniation that does not cause any cord compression on preoperative magnetic resonance (MR) scan. In contrast, **Fig. 1.1B** shows a disk causing moderate cord compression in addition to nerve root compression. The former case would clearly indicate CMED, whereas an anterior decompressive approach would be safer and more effective in the latter case. Whether the pathology is soft disk or hard osteophyte, it must be lateralized and without significant central stenosis for consideration of performing a CMEF/D. In cases of moderate canal stenosis in the presence of normal cervical lordosis, consideration can be given to CMEDS or traditional open laminectomy or laminoplasty.

◆ Operative Technique

General endotracheal anesthesia is induced in the usual fashion. The use of an arterial line, Foley catheter, and evoked potentials is discretionary. A precordial Doppler may be used to monitor for air embolism, though our group has not experienced this complication to date, which we attribute to the low risk of air embolism with a small exposure. The table is then turned 180 degrees relative to the anesthesia workstation. The patient is placed in Mayfield three-point head fixation, and the table is progressively flexed and placed into a Trendelenburg position, which brings the patient into a semisitting posture such that the head is flexed but not rotated and the long axis of the cervical spine is perpendicular to the floor (**Fig. 1.2A–C**). The Mayfield is secured to a table-mounted crossbar, and the patient's arms are folded across the lap or chest depending upon body habitus. The legs, hands, and arms are carefully padded to prevent positional neural injury. The fluoroscopic and endoscopic monitors are placed next to the head of the patient opposite the side of approach, which allows the surgeon to look directly at the monitors while standing behind the patient and operating through the tubular retractor at a comfortable height. The base of the fluoroscopic C-arm is placed on the side ipsilateral to the surgical approach. The C-arm may be arranged below, above, or in front of the patient (**Fig. 1.2A–C**) depending upon the design specifics of the C-arm and operating table, and whether or not anteroposterior (AP) images are desired during the case. Care is taken to ensure that the neck has been safely positioned to allow for adequate jugular venous drainage and airway patency.

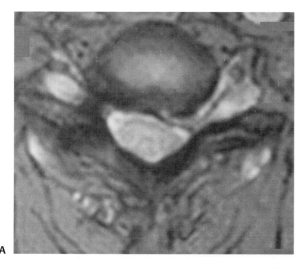

A

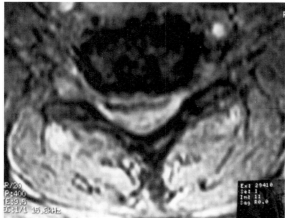

B

Fig. 1.1 Axial T2-weighted cervical spine magnetic resonance imaging scans demonstrate **(A)** a laterally herniated disk to the left with resultant effacement of the lateral thecal sac and compression of the exiting nerve root is ideally suited for the CMEF/D and **(B)** a centrally located disk/osteophyte causing both spinal cord and nerve root compression would be best approached with an anterior decompression.

Alternatively, when using the operative microscope, the surgeon is typically more comfortable with the patient in a prone position. Ideally, the head should still be positioned above the level of the heart to decrease venous pressure. This can be accomplished by flexing the table at the midbreak point and placing the head in a "concorde" position relative to the thorax, with the neck parallel to the floor.

Prior to draping, an initial fluoroscopic image is obtained to confirm adequate visualization and to plan the initial entry point. In the unusual event that the operative level cannot be visualized on lateral fluoroscopy despite positioning changes and

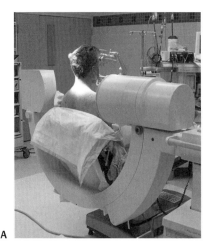
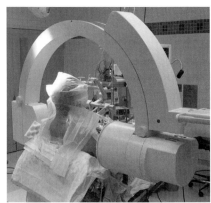

A

B

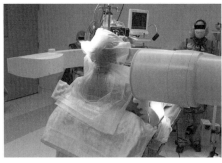

C

Fig. 1.2 Operative positioning of a patient in Mayfield head fixation for cervical microendoscopic foraminotomy/diskectomy or cervical microendoscopic decompression of stenosis with the various positions of the intraoperative fluoroscope C-arm: **(A)** beneath the patient, **(B)** above the patient, and **(C)** in front of the patient.

taping of the shoulders, the procedure should likely be abandoned. The posterior neck is then shaved, scrubbed, prepared, and draped in the usual sterile fashion. Adhesive-lined drapes or an antibacterial adhesive layer, such as Ioban (3M Health Care, St. Paul, MN), or both, are often useful in maintaining the orientation and position of the drapes during the procedure. Suction tubing, cautery lines, the endoscope light source, and camera cables are typically draped over the top or side of the field and secured against the drapes. The operative level is again confirmed on lateral fluoroscopy while a long K-wire or Steinmann pin is held over the lateral side of the patient's neck. An 18 mm longitudinal incision is marked out ~1.5 cm off the midline on the operative side and then injected with local anesthesia. For two-level procedures, the incision should be placed midway between the levels of interest. For bilateral procedures, a midline skin incision can be used and the skin retracted to each side for independent dilations. After an initial stab incision, the K-wire is advanced slowly though the musculature under fluoroscopic guidance and docked at the inferomedial edge of the rostral lateral mass of the level of interest (**Fig. 1.3A**). It is critical to identify and palpate bone and not penetrate the interlaminar space where the laterally thinned ligamentum flavum may not protect against iatrogenic dural or spinal cord injury. At this point the incision is completed ~1 cm rostral and

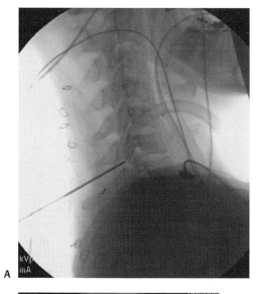

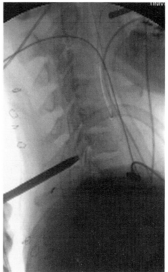

A

B

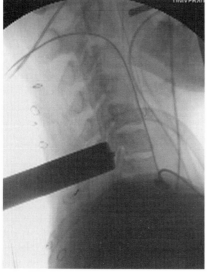

C

Fig. 1.3 Intraoperative lateral fluoroscopic images demonstrating the process of muscle dilation. **(A)** K-wire is docked on the laminofacet junction over the intervertebral foramen of interest (C6–7 in this case). **(B)** The first two muscle dilators are inserted serially. **(C)** Progression to the largest dilator is complete. (*continued*)

caudal to the K-wire entry point and the wire is then removed. The axial forces that are applied during muscle dilation in the lumbar spine are more hazardous in the cervical spine. Therefore, the cervical fascia is incised equal to the length of the incision using monopolar cautery or scissors so that muscle dilation may be performed in a safe and controlled fashion. The K-wire is reinserted under fluoroscopy, and the tubular muscle dilators are serially placed (**Fig. 1.3B–D**). Alternatively, once the fascia is incised, the first dilator, with its relatively blunt end, may be placed instead of

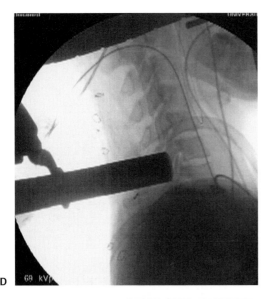

D

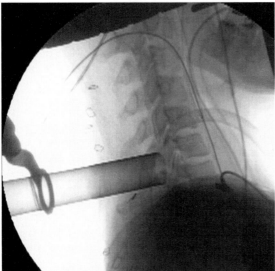

E

Fig. 1.3 (*continued*)　Intraoperative lateral fluoroscopic images demonstrating the process of muscle dilation. **(D)** An 18 mm tubular retractor is placed over the dilators. **(E)** The retractor is fixed into place and dilators are removed.

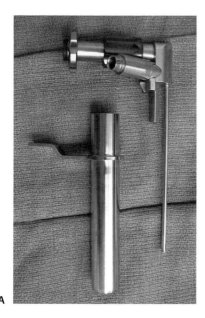
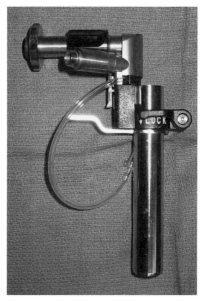

A   B

Fig. 1.4 Photographs of **(A)** METRx tubular retractor (Medtronic Sofamor Danek, Memphis, TN) and rigid 25 degree glass rod endoscope, and **(B)** the endoscope inserted into the tube and fixed in place with a cylindrical plastic friction couple.

the K-wire. After dilation is completed, a final 16 or 18 mm tubular METRx retractor (Medtronic Sofamor Danek, Memphis, TN) is placed over the dilators and fixed into place over the laminofacet junction with a table-mounted retractor arm, and the dilators are removed (**Fig. 1.3E**). A 25 degree angled glass rod endoscope is attached to the camera, white-balanced, and treated with an antifog solution prior to insertion and attachment to the tube via a cylindrical plastic friction-couple (**Fig. 1.4A,B**).

Monopolar cautery and pituitary rongeurs are used to clear the remaining soft tissue off of the lateral mass and lamina of interest, taking care to start the dissection over solid bone laterally (**Fig. 1.5A**). A small up-angled curette is used to gently detach the ligamentum flavum from the undersurface of the inferior edge of the lamina, and a Kerrison punch with a small footplate is used to begin the laminotomy. At this point the CMEF/D and CMEDS diverge in their course. We describe the technique for CMEF/D first, followed by CMEDS.

Cervical Microendoscopic Diskectomy/Foraminotomy: Technique

The subsequent steps of the operation differ little from the open procedure. Depending upon the degree of facet hypertrophy, the Kerrison may be used to complete most of the laminotomy and early foraminotomy, or the drill may be required early in the course of bone removal (**Fig. 1.5B**). The use of a fine cutting bit and adjustable guard sleeve greatly facilitates maneuvering the drill around critical neural structures (**Fig. 1.6A,B**). The ligamentum flavum can be removed medially

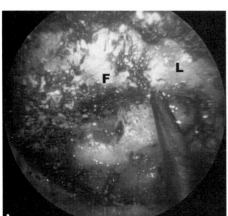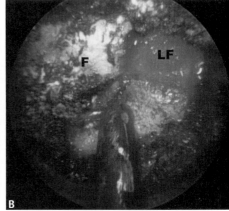

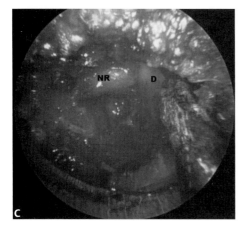

Fig. 1.5 Intraoperative endoscopic photographs during left-sided cervical microendoscopic foraminotomy (CMEF). In all photos, rostral is to the top and medial is to the right. **(A)** Initial exposure reveals lateral edge of lamina (*L*) joining the medial facet (*F*) with a fine upgoing curette inserted under the caudal edge of the laminofacet junction. **(B)** After initial laminotomy, the ligamentum flavum (*LF*) is seen with the adjacent facet (*F*). **(C)** After foraminotomy, the lateral edge of the dura (*D*) and decompressed nerve root (*NR*) in the proximal foramen are revealed.

after the laminotomy to identify the lateral edge of the dura and proximal portion of the nerve root (**Fig. 1.5B,C**). The dorsal bony resection should follow the nerve root into the foramen through a partial, medial facetectomy. To maintain biomechanical integrity, at least 50% of the facet should be preserved.[20] This amount of resection also permits adequate exposure of the root in the foramen. With the root well visualized, a fine angled dissector can be used to palpate the space ventral to the nerve root for osteophytes or disk fragments. Should an osteophyte be present, a down-angled curette may be used to tamp the material further ventrally into the disk space or to fragment it for subsequent removal. In the case of a soft disk herniation, a nerve hook may be passed ventrally and inferiorly to the root to gently tease the fragment away from the nerve for ultimate removal with a pituitary rongeur. In either case, additional drilling of the superomedial quadrant of the caudal pedicle allows greater access to the ventral pathology and obviates the need for excessive nerve root retraction superiorly. Hemostasis is achieved with bipolar cautery, bone wax, and any of a variety of commercially available operative hemostatic agents. A methylprednisolone-soaked pledget may be placed over the root to reduce postoperative inflammation.

Cervical Microendoscopic Decompression of Stenosis: Technique

After completion of the ipsilateral laminotomy, the ligamentum flavum is left in place to protect the dura. The tube is then angled ~45 degrees off the midline such that the endoscope and tube are oriented to visualize the contralateral side. The subligamentous plane beneath the undersurface of the spinous process is gently dissected with a fine curette. The drill with guard sleeve extended (**Fig. 1.6A,B**) is then used to progressively remove the bony undersurface of the spinous process and contralateral lamina across to the contralateral facet. This initial decompression creates a larger working space within which hypertrophied ligament may be safely removed by avoiding any downward pressure on the dura and spinal cord. Dissection and removal of the ligament with curettes and Kerrison rongeurs may now proceed

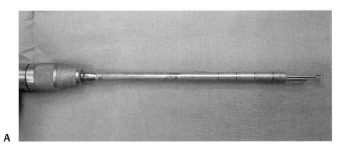

A

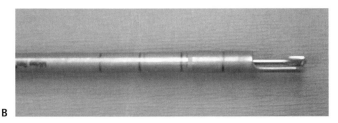

B

Fig. 1.6 Endoscopic drill with TDQ bit (Midas Rex, Fort Worth, TX) and guard sleeve in **(A)** extended and **(B)** retracted positions.

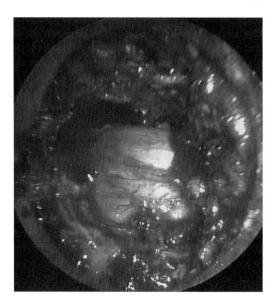

Fig. 1.7 Intraoperative endoscopic photograph during right-sided approach for cervical microendoscopic decompression of stenosis. The dura is seen to be completely decompressed in this image following removal of offending bone and ligament. Rostral is to the right and lateral is to the bottom.

safely. Any compressive elements of the contralateral facet or the superior edge of the caudal lamina may also be drilled off or removed with Kerrison rongeurs at this time because their impact on the dura is more apparent with the ligament removed. A fine probe is gently used to confirm decompression over to the contralateral foramen. The tube is then returned to its original position to complete the ipsilateral removal of ligament and bone. This should then reveal a completely decompressed and pulsatile thecal sac (**Fig. 1.7**). If indicated, ipsilateral foraminotomy as described earlier may be performed at this time as well. The field is irrigated with an antibiotic solution and hemostasis is achieved with bipolar cautery, bone wax, and hemostatic agents. **Figure 1.8A,B** demonstrates a representative case of single-level C4–5 stenosis treated with CMEDS. The typical extent of bony decompression is seen on postoperative CT (**Fig. 1.8C**).

◆ Discussion

The operative indications for a cervical foraminotomy are radiculopathy due to lateral disk herniation or foraminal stenosis (**Fig. 1.1**), persistent or recurrent nerve root symptoms following anterior cervical diskectomy and fusion, and cervical disk disease in patients for whom anterior approaches are relatively contraindicated (anterior neck infection, tracheostomy, prior irradiation, or previous radical neck surgery for neoplasm).[13] Contraindications to CMEF/D include pure axial neck pain without neurological symptoms, gross cervical instability, symptomatic central disk herniation, excessive burden of ventral compression (e.g., diffuse OPLL), or a kyphotic deformity that would render a posterior decompression ineffective and likely destabilize the patient's cervical spine.

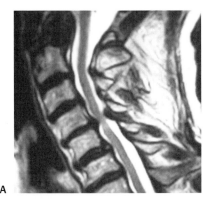
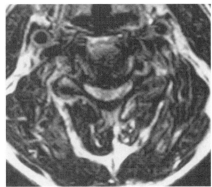

A

B

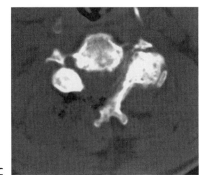

C

Fig. 1.8 An 80-year-old male presented with chronic myelopathy from cervical stenosis and underwent right-sided approach for C4–5 microendoscopic decompression of stenosis (MEDS). **(A)** Sagittal T2-weighted magnetic resonance imaging (MRI) demonstrates focal C4–5 spondylotic stenosis with signal change in the spinal cord. **(B)** Axial T2-weighted MRI reveals severe focal compression at C4–5. **(C)** Postoperative axial computed tomographic image shows typical extent of bony resection required to achieve adequate decompression of the spinal cord. Note the preservation of the dorsal spinous process and contralateral lamina and facet. Also note the minimal impact on paraspinal soft tissues on the approach side (postoperative air is seen on the approach side and at the site of the laminotomy).

Any patient with the aforementioned indications is a candidate for a single-level minimally invasive foraminotomy. The procedure can be performed endoscopically with the patient in the sitting position as described earlier, or with surgical loops or the microscope with the patient in the more traditional prone position with the Mayfield head holder. Placement of the patient in the sitting position is not difficult, even for those surgeons who do not routinely perform surgery in this manner. There is a short learning curve associated with operating while standing and applying instruments through the working channel at the operator's chest level while observing the monitor. The additional advantages of the sitting position are improved visualization within the working channel because of decreased venous bleeding as well as superior radiographic visualization for low cervical or cervicothoracic foraminotomies because of the gravitational effect on the patient's shoulders.[9,13] An open foraminotomy is a reasonable alternative in patients who are very thin with a short skin to facet joint distance (usually less than 4 cm). In these patients, tubular dilation can be difficult and hampered by muscle creep.

A two-level CMEF/D can easily be performed with a single incision and cephalocaudal angulation of the working channel without a significant increase in operative time. A three-level CMEF/D usually requires elongation of the incision and fascia and a second muscular dilation that can prolong the surgery and increase the complication rate, particularly if the patients are placed in the sitting position. If the surgeon does not perform these routinely, we recommend an open multilevel foraminotomy, laminectomy with or without fusion, or laminoplasty for three-level disease.

A cadaveric feasibility study on CMEF/D demonstrated the ability to achieve equivalent bony resection and nerve root decompression when directly compared with traditional open techniques.[21,22] The reports of CMEF/D used clinically[9,13,23] have demonstrated efficacy that is equivalent to traditional open procedures (87–97% rate of symptom relief) but with a marked reduction in blood loss, length of stay, and postoperative pain medication usage in CMEF/D cases.

Our group has recently reviewed clinical outcomes after CMEF/D using validated outcome instruments in a prospective cohort of 30 patients (unpublished data). In these patients, mean visual analog scale (VAS) scores decreased from 2.0 to 0.6 for headache, 5.0 to 2.1 for neck pain, and 4.8 to 1.9 for arm pain. Mean Neck Disability Index scores improved from 37.7 to 20.8, and mean Short Form-36 scores showed statistically significant improvements for bodily pain, physical function, and role physical subscales. Mean operative blood loss was 80 mL, and mean hospital stay for the cohort was 10 hours. When combined with the evidence accumulated in the literature to date, these data establish CMEF/D as a safe, effective, and minimally invasive outpatient procedure for the treatment of isolated cervical radiculopathy.

The indications for CMEDS are central spondylotic stenosis (e.g., ligamentum flavum or facet hypertrophy) in patients presenting with myelopathy or myeloradiculopathy. The neurological symptoms should correlate with radiographic findings. Minimally invasive decompression of the cervical spinal cord can be technically challenging with a potential for disastrous complications. In our opinion, CMEDS should only be performed by the experienced spine surgeon accustomed to performing minimally invasive cervical spine surgery. Like CMEF/D, the procedure can be performed in the sitting or prone position depending on the surgeon's comfort. The ideal candidate is one with significant dorsal disease from ligamentum flavum hypertrophy at one or two levels. Stenosis at three or more levels is best treated with an open decompression with or without fusion or laminoplasty because of the ease and rapidity with which this can be accomplished compared with its minimally invasive counterpart.

The feasibility of minimal access multilevel laminectomy and laminoplasty techniques was also first demonstrated in cadaver models.[24,25] In separate studies, both techniques demonstrated a 43% expansion of the cross-sectional area of the spinal canal.[16,24,25] Clinical application of minimally invasive posterior cervical decompression for stenosis, however, has not been studied as extensively as CMEF/D. The use of minimally invasive cervical laminoplasty has been reported in four patients as technically feasible and safe, with a postoperative mean improvement of 1.25 points on the Nurick scale.[24] The authors of the minimally invasive laminoplasty studies have noted technical difficulties associated with elevation of the lamina and the insertion of bone grafts.

Yabuki and Kikuchi[26] published their series of 10 patients operated upon for cervical spondylotic myelopathy utilizing the endoscopic METRx system (Medtronic Sofamor Danek, Memphis, TN). Using bilateral dilations and laminotomies to remove dorsal bony and ligamentous compression, they treated up to two levels of stenosis and reported a mean operative time of 164 minutes, mean blood loss of 45 mL, and mean posterior neck VAS scores of 2.8 on postoperative day 1 and 0.8 on postoperative day 3.[26] Although no control group was presented, the authors anecdotally felt that the decrease in postoperative neck pain compared with open procedures was dramatic. At a mean follow-up of 15 months, patients had a mean improvement in their Japanese Orthopedic Association score of 2.5 points. The authors reported no complications, instances of postoperative instability, or need for reoperation.[26]

To preserve the contralateral bony and superficial ligamentous structures and to limit the approach to a single muscle dilation, our group prefers a unilateral approach to CMEDS, as described here. Fessler and colleagues have previously reported on five patients undergoing CMEDS at one, two, or three levels.[16] All patients demonstrated improvement in their myelopathy and returned to work, with the only complication being one unintended durotomy that sealed spontaneously.

Typical complication rates from posterior cervical decompressive procedures range from 2 to 9%, with infection and cerebrospinal fluid (CSF) leaks the most common.[9] We have not had any infections in our series to date, and our unintended durotomy rate has dropped from 8% in the initial series of patients[9] to around 1% more recently. Direct suture repair of durotomy is difficult through the narrow-diameter tubes. Therefore, one technique for handling small defects is simply to cover the durotomy with muscle, fat, Gelfoam (Pfizer, New York, NY), or dural substitute followed by fibrin glue or synthetic sealants. Using this approach, overnight bed rest is usually sufficient to seal the defect. For larger dural tears that cannot be primarily closed, 2 to 3 days of lumbar CSF drainage may prevent a leak. Fortunately, the small opening and relative lack of dead space after minimally invasive procedures have made the incidence of postoperative pseudomeningoceles and CSF-cutaneous fistulae negligible.

Potential neurological complications include root injury from manipulation within a tight neural foramen or direct mechanical spinal cord injury during dilation or decompression. Vertebral artery injury can be avoided by early detection of dark venous bleeding from the venous plexus surrounding the artery that may arise from accidental dilation lateral to the facet or during overly aggressive dissection laterally in the foramen. Packing with Gelfoam or other hemostatic agents can typically control venous bleeding. As mentioned previously, despite the use of the semisitting position, air embolism has not presented a problem to date. Delayed complications, such as recurrent disease or postoperative instability, also have not been observed in our use of these techniques thus far.

◆ Conclusion

Posterior CMEF/D and CMEDS offer several benefits: decreased blood loss, markedly reduced length of stay, reduced postoperative pain and muscle spasm, preservation of motion segments, and decreased risk of iatrogenic sagittal plane deformity, while delivering efficacy equivalent to their open counterparts.[9] The appeal of these minimally invasive procedures for degenerative conditions of the cervical spine lies in the reduction of immediate and delayed operative morbidity combined with safe and effective decompression. Spine surgeons should consider an open approach for multilevel disease because of the relative ease and rapidity with which this can be performed compared with its minimally invasive counterpart. As more surgeons become familiar with microendoscopic techniques, their use will likely become more widespread.

References

1. Aldrich F. Posterolateral microdisectomy for cervical monoradiculopathy caused by posterolateral soft cervical disc sequestration. J Neurosurg 1990;72:370–377

2. Crandall PH, Batzdorf U. Cervical spondylotic myelopathy. J Neurosurg 1966;25:57–66

3. Henderson CM, Hennessy RG, Shuey HM Jr, Shackelford EG. Posterior-lateral foraminotomy as an exclusive operative technique for cervical radiculopathy: a review of 846 consecutively operated cases. Neurosurgery 1983;13:504–512

4. Ratliff JK, Cooper PR. Cervical laminoplasty: a critical review. J Neurosurg 2003;98(3, Suppl): 230–238

5. Khoo LT, Perez-Cruet MJ, Laich DT, Fessler RG. Posterior cervical microendoscopic foraminotomy. In: Perez-Cruet MJ, Fessler RG, eds. Outpatient Spinal Surgery. St. Louis, MO: Quality Medical Publishing; 2006:71–93

6. Kumar VG, Rea GL, Mervis LJ, McGregor JM. Cervical spondylotic myelopathy: functional and radiographic long-term outcome after laminectomy and posterior fusion. Neurosurgery 1999; 44:771–777

7. Wang MY, Green BA. Laminoplasty for the treatment of failed anterior cervical spine surgery. Neurosurg Focus 2003;15:E7

8. Wang MY, Shah S, Green BA. Clinical outcomes following cervical laminoplasty for 204 patients with cervical spondylotic myelopathy. Surg Neurol 2004;62:487–492

9. Fessler RG, Khoo LT. Minimally invasive cervical microendoscopic foraminotomy: an initial clinical experience. Neurosurgery 2002;51(5, Suppl):S37–S45

10. Hilibrand AS, Robbins M. Adjacent segment degeneration and adjacent segment disease: the consequences of spinal fusion? Spine J 2004;4(6, Suppl):190S–194S

11. Ishihara H, Kanamori M, Kawaguchi Y, Nakamura H, Kimura T. Adjacent segment disease after anterior cervical interbody fusion. Spine J 2004;4:624–628

12. Hosono N, Yonenobu K, Ono K. Neck and shoulder pain after laminoplasty: a noticeable complication. Spine (Phila Pa 1976) 1996;21:1969–1973

13. Siddiqui A, Yonemura KS. Posterior cervical microendoscopic diskectomy and laminoforaminotomy. In: Kim DH, Fessler RG, Regan JJ, eds. Endoscopic Spine Surgery and Instrumentation: Percutaneous Procedures. New York: Thieme; 2005:66–73

14. Albert TJ, Vacarro A. Postlaminectomy kyphosis. Spine (Phila Pa 1976) 1998;23:2738–2745

15. Kaptain GJ, Simmons NE, Replogle RE, Pobereskin L. Incidence and outcome of kyphotic deformity following laminectomy for cervical spondylotic myelopathy. J Neurosurg 2000;93(2, Suppl):199–204

16. Perez-Cruet MJ, Samartzis D, Fessler RG. Microendoscopic cervical laminectomy. In: Perez-Cruet MJ, Khoo LT, Fessler RG, eds. An Anatomic Approach to Minimally Invasive Spine Surgery. St. Louis, MO: Quality Medical Publishing; 2006:16–11–16–17.

17. Yonenobu K, Okada K, Fuji T, Fujiwara K, Yamashita K, Ono K. Causes of neurologic deterioration following surgical treatment of cervical myelopathy. Spine (Phila Pa 1976) 1986;11:818–823

18. Khoo LT, Bresnahan L, Fessler RG. Cervical endoscopic foraminotomy. In: Fessler RG, Sekhar L, eds. Atlas of Neurosurgical Techniques: Spine and Peripheral Nerves. Vol 1. New York: Thieme; 2006:785–792

19. Khoo LT, Fessler RG. Microendoscopic decompressive laminotomy for the treatment of lumbar stenosis. Neurosurgery 2002;51(5, Suppl):S146–S154

20. Raynor RB, Pugh J, Shapiro I. Cervical facetectomy and its effect on spine strength. J Neurosurg 1985;63:278–282

21. Burke TG, Caputy A. Microendoscopic posterior cervical foraminotomy: a cadaveric model and clinical application for cervical radiculopathy. J Neurosurg 2000;93(1, Suppl):126–129

22. Roh SW, Kim DH, Cardoso AC, Fessler RG. Endoscopic foraminotomy using MED system in cadaveric specimens. Spine (Phila Pa 1976) 2000;25:260–264

23. Adamson TE. Microendoscopic posterior cervical laminoforaminotomy for unilateral radiculopathy: results of a new technique in 100 cases. J Neurosurg 2001;95(1, Suppl):51–57

24. Perez-Cruet MJ, Wang MY, Samartzis D. Microendoscopic cervical laminectomy and laminoplasty. In: Kim DH, Fessler RG, Regan JJ, eds. Endoscopic Spine Surgery and Instrumentation: Percutaneous Procedures. New York: Thieme; 2005:74–87

25. Wang MY, Green BA, Coscarella E, Baskaya MK, Levi AD, Guest JD. Minimally invasive cervical expansile laminoplasty: an initial cadaveric study. Neurosurgery 2003;52:370–373

26. Yabuki S, Kikuchi S. Endoscopic partial laminectomy for cervical myelopathy. J Neurosurg Spine 2005;2:170–174

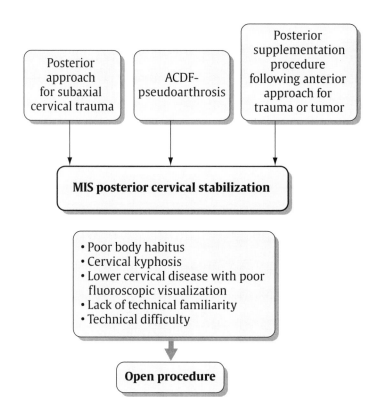

2

Posterior Cervical Fixation

Rikin A. Trivedi and Michael Y. Wang

Advances in digital fluoroscopy, image guidance systems, and surgical endoscopy have improved intraoperative visualization such that a wide range of surgeries can now be performed through smaller incisions. Such approaches result in less local tissue damage, blood loss, and reduced overall morbidity. Because traditional open posterior approaches to the cervical spine necessitate extensive subperiosteal dissection and muscular retraction, they can be associated with increased intraoperative blood loss and prolonged postoperative pain. Thus these approaches in particular may be improved through the application of minimally invasive surgical (MIS) techniques.

In open posterior cervical surgery the extent of dissection required and subperiosteal muscle and ligamentous stripping are far in excess of the exposure needed at the target area for decompression or instrumentation. Although these factors have driven the evolution of more minimally invasive techniques, such approaches need to meet certain predetermined criteria. First, the minimally invasive approach must have an equivalent or superior safety profile. Second, it must be as effective as the open procedure. Third, the procedure must be easily adoptable by the surgical community at large. Fourth, it must be cost-effective and not require excessive capital equipment or implant expenditures.

Numerous publications already suggest that several minimally invasive spinal surgeries have already fulfilled these criteria. Microscopic posterior cervical foraminotomy has long been an effective procedure for treating cervical radiculopathy through foraminal unroofing and disk/osteophyte removal,[1-4] but the success of this procedure was often affected by significant postoperative cervicalgia and muscle spasm. The advent of microendoscopic laminoforaminotomy (MELF) allowed the same decompressive surgery to be performed through smaller incisions, with less musculoligamentous disruption[5-15] through the use of a series of tubular dilator retractors, which were directed over a guide wire placed with the aid of fluoroscopy.

Several different tubular retractor systems are now commercially available and offer versatility while remaining relatively inexpensive, and these systems have become the workhorses of MIS spinal procedures. Utilized in conjunction with intraoperative imaging, frameless navigation, electrophysiological guidance, and microscopic or endoscopic visualization, they provide direct access to the skeletal structures, splitting the muscle fibers over it rather than cutting them. Using a tubular dilator system, the path created to the lamina-facet region can be easily redirected so that the access corridor is centered over the cervical lateral masses.

An MIS approach has also been utilized with some success in cadavers and humans for atlantoaxial fixation with transarticular screws or C1 lateral mass/C2 pars screw–rod constructs. This latter strategy was used to treat a patient with C1–2 instability from os odontoideum (**Fig. 2.1**). Early fusion at the C1–2 joint was reported, and the patient was reported to be asymptomatic at 3 months.[16] A tubular dilator system has not been used for C1–2 transarticular fixation; however, image-guided percutaneous instrumentation has been employed in cadavers.[17] Although attractive at the investigational stage, no clinical applications of this have been described. The reason for this perhaps relates to the need to lessen the rotational instability that a C1–2 transarticular screw does not satisfactorily address as well as achieve bony fusion. Additionally, the margin of safety may also be a concern, given the narrow portal.

Subaxial cervical lateral mass screw constructs have been successfully utilized for posterior cervical fusion and fixation. Depending on the patient's physique, up to three adjacent lateral masses can be easily accessed using a 16 to 22 mm working port through a single midline incision. The ergonomic screw trajectory through a midline approach, combined with the robust safety of this technique and favorable fusion environment, have made this a clinically feasible technique. To date, several groups have successfully used such tubular portals to perform both screw–plate and screw–rod fixation in the subaxial spine and have achieved excellent clinical and radiographic results.[18–21]

The minimally invasive posterior stabilization procedure can be performed for the same indications as an open procedure, including trauma, infection, malignant disease, and spondylitic disease.[22] Caution should be exercised in cases with significant kyphosis due to the distant screw entry sites, limited ability to compress across screw heads, and rod lengths required. Furthermore, screw–plate constructs, unlike the screw–rod constructs, will only allow in situ stabilization and no reduction of the kyphosis. In general, the technique for screw insertion does not differ significantly from the open technique, allowing application of the specific methods advocated by Roy-Camille, Magerl, or An.[23–25] In both open and MIS cases, a trajectory path guided cephalad avoids neural injury, and a path guided laterally minimizes the risk of vascular injury. The lengths of screws employed are also similar to when the open technique is used (12 to 16 mm) and will vary depending on bony morphology, trajectory and starting point.

◆ Preoperative Evaluation

The mainstay of preoperative planning is the radiographic examination, which should include plain films performed in neutral, flexion, and extension. This will identify segmental instability and significant kyphosis, both of which may contraindicate a posterior approach. A CT of the cervical spine is useful in outlining the bony

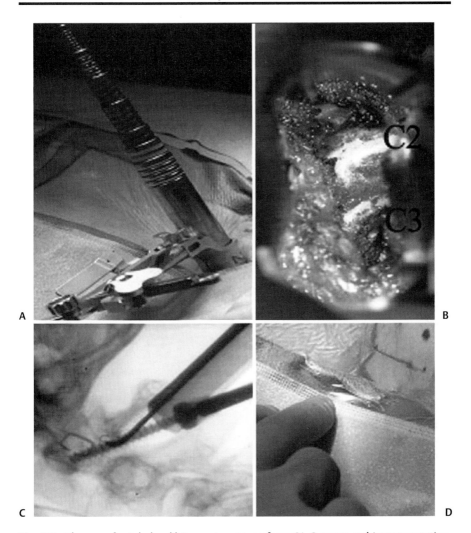

Fig. 2.1 The use of a tubular dilator system to perform C1–2 screw–rod instrumentation. **(A)** Sequential insertion of the tubular dilators. **(B)** Exposure provided at the end of the dilation process. **(C)** Insertion of a C1 lateral mass screw through the working portal. **(D)** Paramedian incision after one side is completed. (From Joseffer SS, Post N, Cooper PR, Frempong-Boadu AK. Minimally invasive atlanto-axial fixation with a polyaxial screw-rod construct: technical case report. Neurosurgery 2006;58(4, Suppl 2):E375. Reprinted with permission.)

anatomy of the lateral mass and facet joints better as well as allowing preoperative determination of screw length. MRI is useful for delineating any associated soft tissue abnormalities and for assessing the extent of any coexistent neural impingement.

◆ Operative Technique

General anesthesia is preferable to local anesthesia and intravenous sedation because of the imminent risk to the neurovascular structure with intraoperative patient movement. The Mayfield head clamp is then applied and used to provide rigid fixation in the prone position. Intraoperative electrophysiological monitoring can be useful to assess the integrity of the nerve roots and spinal cord by using somatosensory evoked potential (SSEP) monitoring, and electromyographic (EMG) and motor evoked potential (MEP) recordings. The patient is then positioned prone, with the table manipulated so that the head is above the heart to reduce venous engorgement and blood loss. The neck posture is then adjusted according to the pathology treated, but the Mayfield attachment should remain accessible so that intraoperative manipulation to place the neck into physiological lordosis prior to rod placement can be accomplished. Adhesive tape is then used to retract the shoulders, especially if visualization of the lower cervical spine will be required, as fluoroscopic C-arm images will be critical to guide hardware implantation. Prior to skin incision, lateral images should be taken to ensure that all relevant lateral masses are visible. In some instances the sitting position can be advantageous to keep the shoulders out of the field of imaging, to allow instrumentation of lower levels.

A Steinmann pin is positioned lateral to the neck with an inclination such that it parallels the orientation of the facet joint between the target lateral masses. The skin incision is then marked accordingly on or just medial to the midline. It will be noticed that the skin incision is several spinal segments caudad of the lateral masses to be instrumented, but the trajectory afforded by this skin incision is similar to that in open cases. Using fluoroscopic guidance, the Steinmann pin is inserted through the fascia and cervical musculature down to the level of the facet joint and adjacent lateral masses. The trajectory of the pin is in a superior and lateral direction (akin to the desired trajectory of the lateral mass screw). Great care should be exercised not to introduce the pin into the interlaminar space or lateral to the vertebrae because this has been observed as a complication of improper technique or inadequate use of fluoroscopy. Anteroposterior (AP) fluoroscopy can be used to confirm the ideal docking site of the pin, which is at the medial aspect of the facet complex. Alternatively, after the appropriate trajectory has been determined, a full 2 cm skin incision can be made in the midline with an accompanying fascial incision. This allows docking onto the lateral masses with the smallest introducer tube, limiting the likelihood of iatrogenic injury (**Fig. 2.2**).

Once satisfactory docking has occurred, the skin incision should be extended equally in the rostral–caudal plane to avoid skin necrosis from the subsequent introduction of the dilators. If an adhesive drape has been used, then a sufficiently sized window is needed to avoid this being introduced into the wound. The underlying cervical fascia should also be opened to facilitate the sequential insertion of tubular dilators, but the extent of this need not be as long as the skin opening. Care should be taken to avoid cutting into the muscle because this is a cause of unnecessary

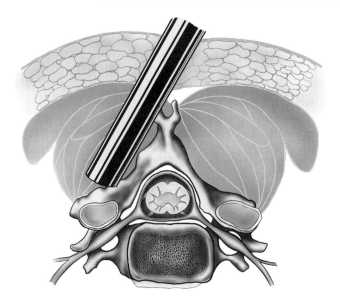

Fig. 2.2 The site of docking of the tubular retractor system is at the facet joint complex in a trajectory planned for screw insertion.

bleeding. The dilators are then sequentially passed over one another to progressively enlarge the working channel. Each dilator should be inserted to a depth that anchors it to the bony surface, and this can be confirmed as often as is required by lateral fluoroscopy. The final tube diameter will depend upon the number of levels treated as well as the patient's body size. Tubes with a conical shape can also be used to limit the length of the skin incision while maximizing the working corridor. Once the length and diameter of the working portal are determined, this retractor is inserted and attached to a flexible retractor arm, which is fixed to the opposite side of the operating table (**Fig. 2.3**). Lateral fluoroscopy is used to ensure correct docking and trajectory before final tightening of the flexible retractor arm-portal connection.

At this stage a decision can be made as to whether the endoscope is to be used; if it is, then this can be mounted onto the working portal either directly or via a coupler, depending on which access system is used. Direct inspection down the working portal using either surgical loupes or fiberoptic cable for illumination is also appropriate. The bony surface of the lateral mass and the intervening facet joints should then be exposed by removing overlying soft tissue with monopolar cautery and a pituitary rongeur. Care should be taken, however, not to disrupt the facet complexes above and below the target level so as to avoid inadvertent adjacent-level instability or fusion. The joint and surrounding lateral mass are then decorticated with a high-speed drill to prepare the host fusion bed.

For cases involving a facet dislocation that has not been successfully reduced preoperatively, the superior articular facet of the inferior lateral mass can then be drilled off using a high-speed burr, allowing for easy reduction by repositioning of the Mayfield skull clamp into neck extension. Another option would be to insert a blunt

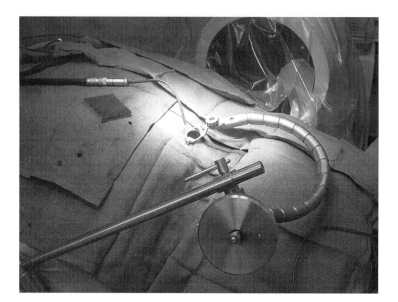

Fig. 2.3 The final working portal is then held rigidly in place using a flexible retractor arm; visualization is improved by the use of an endoscope or fiberoptic light source.

tip instrument such as a Swedish or Penfield into the joint and rotate it such that it reduces the subluxed superior lateral mass by bringing it up and posteriorly. The use of SSEP monitoring ensures that this maneuver can be performed safely. The entry points for lateral mass screw insertion are then created with the high-speed drill. We typically mark an entry point 1 mm medial to the midpoint of the lateral mass. We then pack the joints to be fused with bony dust saved from the drilling, autograft, or allograft because placement of the instrumentation will obstruct the view of the fusion bed later. All of the fusion and instrumentation is accomplished on one side prior to proceeding with the other side.

Screw insertion is then undertaken as per the open procedure and is guided by lateral fluoroscopy. Typically, a pneumatic trauma drill is used, but a hand-driven drill can be used to drill between 12 to 16 mm into the lateral mass in an upward and lateral trajectory, similar to the orientation and trajectory of the working portal (**Fig. 2.4**). The usual screw diameter is either 3.5 or 4.0 mm, and most modern systems have screws with polyaxial heads that are self-tapping. The screw is then inserted along the same trajectory (**Fig. 2.5**). Once the first screw is placed, if a rigid tubular retractor system is being used, to achieve satisfactory screw insertion, the working portal may have to be repositioned. This can be accomplished by loosening the working portal as before, and then gently lifting it dorsally, above the screw head and reorienting it under direct vision. Care must be taken not to lift it off excessively because soft tissue can creep under the skirts of the tube and obscure satisfactory bony docking. This maneuver may not need to be performed for single-level fusions because both lateral masses may be adequately visualized, or with two-level fusions, using an expandable tubular port system. The subsequent screw is then placed as already described.

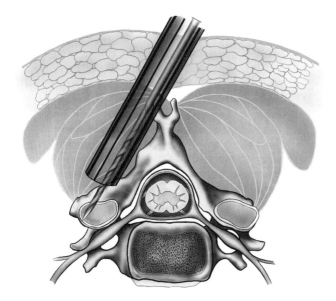

Fig. 2.4 The trajectory of the drill is in line with the working portal, and similar to the open procedure, being directed cephalad and laterally.

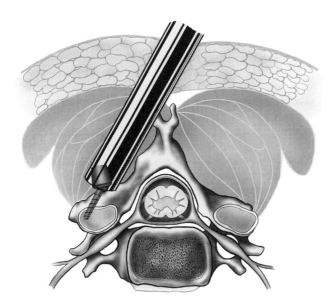

Fig. 2.5 The screw is then inserted through the working portal along the same trajectory.

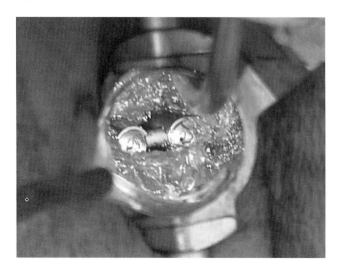

Fig. 2.6 An appropriately sized rod is then passed onto the screw heads and secured with screw caps.

An appropriately sized rod is then selected for insertion and passed down the working portal and manipulated into one of the top-loading polyaxial screw heads (**Fig. 2.6**). If both screw heads are visible through the working portal, then the rod can be translated rostral/caudal into the other screw head. If they are not both visible or if two levels are being fused, then lifting it off the working portal and re-angling it, as earlier described for the screw insertion, will be required. Once again, this requires care to avoid soft tissue prolapse into the working channel. Once the rod is correctly applied it can be secured in place with the locking set screw. Care must be taken to avoid cross-threading this junction, which is prone to happen given the inability to visualize the articulation from laterally. Satisfactory positioning of the instrumentation should then be confirmed with both lateral and AP fluoroscopy. The identical sequence of steps can then be undertaken to perform the contralateral instrumentation prior to retractor removal and wound closure. A wound drain is not required due to the small size of the wound. The wound is then closed in a standard multilayered fashion with resorbable sutures. Local anesthetic can be infiltrated to minimize the postoperative discomfort, and Dermabond (Ethicon, Inc., Somerville, NJ) can be applied to the skin to supplement the skin closure.

◆ Discussion

Our clinical experience of minimally invasive posterior cervical stabilization consists of 18 patients, all of whom had lateral mass screw–rod constructs inserted as part of the treatment for cervical spine trauma, infection, pseudarthrosis, and malignant disease. In 14 patients, lateral mass screws were inserted to augment an antecedent anterior cervical decompression and fusion (**Table 2.1**). A total of 39 levels were instrumented, with 16 of 18 patients undergoing successful screw placement

Table 2.1

	Age	Sex	Mechanism	Musculoskeletal Pathology	Neurological Injury	Anterior Surgery	Posterior Levels Treated	Reduction	Unilateral or Bilateral	Graft	Complications	Outcome	Hospital Stay	Blood Loss
1	32	M	MVA	C4/5 fracture subluxation w/ unilateral facet fracture	C5 root entrapment	C4/5 ACDF	C4, C5	Traction	Unilateral	ICBG	None	C5 root improved	2	50
2	56	F	MVA	C3/4 fracture subluxation w/ unilateral facet fracture	Brown Séquard	C3/4 ACDF	C3, C4	Traction	Unilateral	ICBG	None	Neurologically improved	6	70
3	33	M	Diving	Bilateral jumped facets	None	None	C3, C4	Traction	Bilateral	ICBG	None	Intact	2	50
4	58	F	None	Metastatic tumor	None	C4 corpectomy	C3–5	N/A	Unilateral	ICBG	None	Reduced neck pain	3	100
5	18	F	MVA	Burst fracture	None	C5 corpectomy	C4–6	Traction	Bilateral	Corpectomy bone	None	Intact	3	200
6	32	M	None	Pseudarthrosis	None	C5 corpectomy	C4–6	N/A	Bilateral	ICBG	None	Reduced neck pain	2	50
7	44	M	MVA	Burst fracture	Complete quadriplegia	C5 corpectomy	C4–6	N/A	Bilateral	ICBG	Conversion to open surgery for C6 screws	Complete quadriplegia	5	200
8	52	M	Fall	Fracture dislocation	Complete quadriplegia	C5/6 ACDF	C5, C6	Traction	Bilateral	Vertebral body bone	None	Complete quadriplegia	6	150
9	39	F	None	Pseudarthrosis	None	C4/5 ACDF	C4–6	N/A	Bilateral	ICBG	None	Reduced neck pain	1	25
10	37	F	Fall	Unilateral jumped facet	None	None	C4, C5	Intraoperative	Unilateral	ICBG	None	Reduced neck pain	2	35
11	25	M	MVA	Unilateral jumped facet	None	None	C5, C6	Intraoperative	Unilateral	ICBG	Superficial wound infection	Reduced neck pain	3	25
12	33	F	None	Pseudarthrosis	None	C5/6 ACDF	C5, C6	N/A	Bilateral	ICBG	None	No reduction in neck pain	3	40
13	57	F	None	Pseudarthrosis	None	C3/4 ACDF	C5, C6	N/A	Unilateral	ICBG	Iliac crest donor site pain	Reduced neck pain	2	40
14	40	M	Fall	Fracture dislocation	Incomplete quadriplegia	None	C5, C6	Traction	Bilateral	ICBG	None	Incomplete quadriplegia	3	90
15	55	F	None	Metastatic tumor	Myelopathy	C5 corpectomy	C4–6	N/A	Bilateral	ICBG	None	Neurologically improved	1	160
16	72	F	Spondylotic myelopathy	Osteoporosis	Myelopathy	C6 corpectomy	C5–7	N/A	Bilateral	Corpectomy bone	None	Myelopathy improved	2	90
17	36	F	None	Vertebral osteomyelitis	None	C5 corpectomy	C4–6	N/A	Bilateral	ICBG	None	Neurologically intact	14	250
18	22	M	Fall	Burst fracture	Complete quadriplegia	C6 corpectomy	C5–7	N/A	Bilateral	Corpectomy bone	Conversion to open surgery for C7 screws	Complete quadriplegia	7	400

Abbreviations: ACDF, anterior cervical diskectomy and fusion; ICBG, iliac crest bone graft.

(without unintended breaches on CT). In two patients, the minimally invasive procedure had to be abandoned[22] because of inadequate fluoroscopic visualization in the lower cervical spine. Both patients had a large body habitus. In all cases, there was successful fusion confirmed by both CT and dynamic x-rays (**Fig. 2.7A,B**).

There have been other reports of minimally invasive posterior cervical stabilization utilizing both screw–rod[26] and screw–plate systems.[19] These surgeries were performed for several indications: as augmenting stabilization to anterior cervical diskectomy and fusion (ACDF) for traumatic single- and two-level facet subluxations, as stand-alone reduction/stabilization for single- and two-level traumatic facet subluxations, and as posterior augmentation for anterior corpectomy and fusion for neoplasia. In all cases reported, there were no technical failures, and these authors also reported successful fusion at the treated levels as determined by lack of movement on dynamic x-rays and new bone formation on computed tomography (CT). There was only one instance of a misplaced screw, where there was minor breach of the lateral cortex of the C6 lateral mass. There were no treatment complications and no worsening neurological deficits noted.

Should instrumentation be required at the C7 level, several anatomical factors must be considered. First, the lateral mass is much thinner and smaller than that of the more cephalad vertebral body lateral masses. This can make placement of a lateral mass screw technically difficult. However, because there is no vertebral artery in the foramen transversarium at this level, placement of the screw into the pedicle of C7 can be undertaken relatively safely. If the latter option is selected, then one must bear in mind that the medialized screw trajectory will be different from the orientation of the working portal. A small laminotomy of C6–7 can be performed to help palpate and visualize the medial wall of the pedicle to safely aid the cannulation process.

There are specific anatomical considerations to be appreciated with regard to C1–2 instrumentation. First, the course of the vertebral artery can be considerably varied at this level, which makes it more vulnerable to injury; however, given that the artery is most vulnerable to injury at the superior border of the C1 lamina, a paramedian MIS approach would avoid exposing this region. Second, the superior and inferior articular facets of C2 have differing orientations with the corresponding facets of the adjacent lateral masses and are connected by a long, thin, inclining pars/pedicle. This may necessitate the use of an expandable tubular retractor system to visualize both screw entry points. The third consideration is the C2 nerve root; this large nerve root traverses behind the C1–2 facet complex, which makes it prone to injury from the Steinmann pin during the initial docking process. However, the sacrifice of this root, as was described in the original report of open C1–2 posterior stabilization with a rod–plate construct, appears to have no clinically significant morbidity.[27] While MIS C1–2 fusion is technically feasible, it should only be performed in very select cases and in experienced hands. An open posterior C1–2 fusion is most appropriate in patients with severed atlanto-axial instability or at high risk of pseudoarthrosis.

There are distinct advantages in performing a posterior minimally invasive approach to instrumenting and fusing the cervical spine. Biomechanically, the avoidance of aggressive dissection of the posterior neck muscles (trapezius, semispinalis cervicis, multifidus) and ligaments ensures that the integrity of the posterior tension band is maintained.[28,29] Due to the fact that the incision is smaller and access is directed specifically to the target area by a muscle splitting rather than cutting,

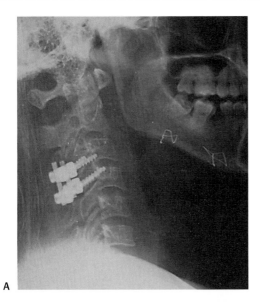

A

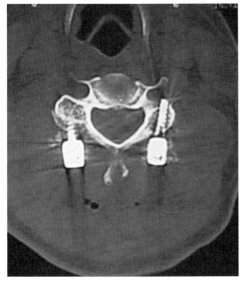

B

Fig. 2.7 (A) Postoperative plain radiograph and (B) axial computed tomography showing satisfactory hardware placement and bone formation at the facet joint complex.

there is less chance of significant postoperative pain, muscle spasm, and disability. Anecdotal reports have also provided evidence for reduced infection rates with the minimally invasive approach.

Despite these advantages, there are some limitations of minimally invasive posterior cervical stabilization: by the very nature of the surgery, the surgeon needs to quickly become familiar with working through a narrow corridor. Coupled with this is the need for the surgeon to become less reliant on direct visualization of the regional anatomy and become more comfortable with two-dimensional visualization using fluoroscopy. There are also some technical limitations: application of the rod to the screw heads can be challenging, particularly when one is fusing multiple spinal segments.

Finally, those patients with morbid obesity and poor body habitus are not good candidates for MIS posterior cervical fixation, given the difficulty in obtaining adequate fluoroscopic visualization, particularly at lower cervical levels.

◆ Conclusion

Instrumentation and fusion of the cervical spine are important parts of the treatment algorithm for several different cervical spine pathologies. The decision to embark upon an anterior or posterior approach is based on several factors, one of which is the degree of iatrogenic damage caused to achieve the ultimate goal of stabilization. Minimally invasive techniques have been well described for neural decompression and stabilization of the lumbar spine.[6,11,12,14,15] More recently minimally invasive techniques have been applied to similar pathologies in the cervical spine via anterior[30-32] and posterior approaches.[5,7-9,26] Surgeons should consider a minimally invasive posterior cervical stabilization procedure for treating pathologies in the subaxial cervical spine. Overall, it is likely that as familiarity with minimally invasive procedures grows, the use of a minimally invasive approach for posterior cervical stabilization is also likely to be increasingly used.

References

1. Grieve JP, Kitchen ND, Moore AJ, Marsh HT. Results of posterior cervical foraminotomy for treatment of cervical spondylitic radiculopathy. Br J Neurosurg 2000;14:40–43

2. Kumar GR, Maurice-Williams RS, Bradford R. Cervical foraminotomy: an effective treatment for cervical spondylotic radiculopathy. Br J Neurosurg 1998;12:563–568

3. Henderson CM, Hennessy RG, Shuey HM Jr, Shackelford EG. Posterior-lateral foraminotomy as an exclusive operative technique for cervical radiculopathy: a review of 846 consecutively operated cases. Neurosurgery 1983;13:504–512

4. Murphey F, Simmons JC, Brunson B. Surgical treatment of laterally ruptured cervical disc: review of 648 cases, 1939 to 1972. J Neurosurg 1973;38:679–683

5. Fessler RG, Khoo LT. Minimally invasive cervical microendoscopic foraminotomy: an initial clinical experience. Neurosurgery 2002;51(5, Suppl):S37–S45

6. Fessler RG, O'Toole JE, Eichholz KM, Perez-Cruet MJ. The development of minimally invasive spine surgery. Neurosurg Clin N Am 2006;17:401–409

7. Holly LT, Moftakhar P, Khoo LT, Wang JC, Shamie N. Minimally invasive 2-level posterior cervical foraminotomy: preliminary clinical results. J Spinal Disord Tech 2007;20:20–24

8. O'Toole JE, Sheikh H, Eichholz KM, Fessler RG, Perez-Cruet MJ. Endoscopic posterior cervical foraminotomy and discectomy. Neurosurg Clin N Am 2006;17:411–422

9. Roh SW, Kim DH, Cardoso AC, Fessler RG. Endoscopic foraminotomy using MED system in cadaveric specimens. Spine (Phila Pa 1976) 2000;25:260–264

10. Perez-Cruet MJ, Fessler RG, Perin NI. Review: complications of minimally invasive spinal surgery. Neurosurgery 2002;51(5, Suppl):S26–S36

11. Fessler RG. Minimally invasive percutaneous posterior lumbar interbody fusion. Neurosurgery 2003;52:1512

12. Guiot BH, Khoo LT, Fessler RG. A minimally invasive technique for decompression of the lumbar spine. Spine (Phila Pa 1976) 2002;27:432–438

13. Isaacs RE, Podichetty VK, Santiago P, et al. Minimally invasive microendoscopy-assisted transforaminal lumbar interbody fusion with instrumentation. J Neurosurg Spine 2005;3:98–105

14. Khoo LT, Fessler RG. Microendoscopic decompressive laminotomy for the treatment of lumbar stenosis. Neurosurgery 2002;51(5, Suppl):S146–S154

15. Sandhu FA, Santiago P, Fessler RG, Palmer S. Minimally invasive surgical treatment of lumbar synovial cysts. Neurosurgery 2004;54:107–111

16. Joseffer SS, Post N, Cooper PR, Frempong-Boadu AK. Minimally invasive atlantoaxial fixation with a polyaxial screw-rod construct: technical case report. Neurosurgery 2006;58(4, Suppl 2):E375

17. Holly LT, Foley KT. Percutaneous placement of posterior cervical screws using three-dimensional fluoroscopy. Spine (Phila Pa 1976) 2006;31:536–540

18. Wang MY, Prusmack CJ, Green BA, Gruen JP, Levi AD. Minimally invasive lateral mass screws in the treatment of cervical facet dislocations: technical note. Neurosurgery 2003;52:444–447

19. Fong S, Duplessis S. Minimally invasive lateral mass plating in the treatment of posterior cervical trauma: surgical technique. J Spinal Disord Tech 2005;18:224–228

20. Khoo LT. Cervical minimally-invasive spinal surgical techniques. In: Annual Meeting of AAISMS, 4th Global Congress on Minimally Invasive Spinal Surgery and Medicine. 2003. Thousand Oaks, CA.

21. Khoo LT. Minimally invasive posterior decompression and fixation of cervical jumped facets: an initial clinical experience in 11 patients. In: Annual Meeting of AANS/CNS Section on Disorders of the Spine and Peripheral Nerves; 2003; Tampa, FL

22. Wang MY, Levi AD. Minimally invasive lateral mass screw fixation in the cervical spine: initial clinical experience with long-term follow-up. Neurosurgery 2006;58:907–912

23. An HS. Internal fixation of the cervical spine: current indications and techniques. J Am Acad Orthop Surg 1995;3:194–206

24. An HS, Gordin R, Renner K. Anatomic considerations for plate-screw fixation of the cervical spine. Spine (Phila Pa 1976) 1991;16(10, Suppl):S548–S551

25. Magerl F, Seeman P, Grob D. Stable dorsal fusion of the cervical spine (C2–T1) using hook plates. In: WA Kehr, ed. Cervical Spine. New York: Springer-Verlag; 1987:217–221

26. Wang MY, Green BA, Coscarella E, Baskaya MK, Levi AD, Guest JD. Minimally invasive cervical expansile laminoplasty: an initial cadaveric study. Neurosurgery 2003;52:370–373

27. Goel A, Laheri V. Plate and screw fixation for atlanto-axial subluxation. Acta Neurochir (Wien) 1994;129:47–53

28. Jahng TA, Fu TS, Cunningham BW, Dmitriev AE, Kim DH. Endoscopic instrumented posterolateral lumbar fusion with Healos and recombinant human growth/differentiation factor-5. Neurosurgery 2004;54:171–180

29. Kim DY, Lee SH, Chung SK, Lee HY. Comparison of multifidus muscle atrophy and trunk extension muscle strength: percutaneous versus open pedicle screw fixation. Spine (Phila Pa 1976) 2005;30:123–129

30. Rubino F, Deutsch H, Pamoukian V, Zhu JF, King WA, Gagner M. Minimally invasive spine surgery: an animal model for endoscopic approach to the anterior cervical and upper thoracic spine. J Laparoendosc Adv Surg Tech A 2000;10:309–313

31. Saringer WF, Reddy B, Nöbauer-Huhmann I, et al. Endoscopic anterior cervical foraminotomy for unilateral radiculopathy: anatomical morphometric analysis and preliminary clinical experience. J Neurosurg 2003;98(2, Suppl):171–180

32. Tan J, Zheng Y, Gong L, Liu X, Li J, Du W. Anterior cervical discectomy and interbody fusion by endoscopic approach: a preliminary report. J Neurosurg Spine 2008;8:17–21

Section II

Thoracic Spine

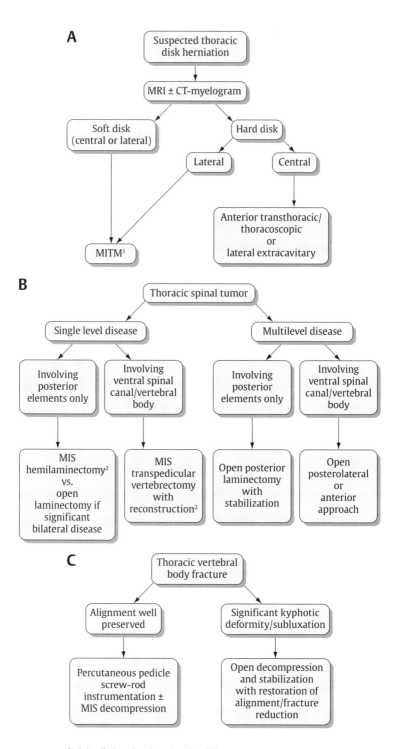

A

Suspected thoracic
disk herniation

↓

MRI ± CT-myelogram

Soft disk
(central or lateral)

Hard disk

Lateral

Central

Anterior transthoracic/
thoracoscopic
or
lateral extracavitary

MITM[1]

B

Thoracic spinal tumor

Single level disease

Multilevel disease

Involving
posterior
elements only

Involving
ventral spinal
canal/vertebral
body

Involving
posterior
elements only

Involving
ventral spinal
canal/vertebral
body

MIS
hemilaminectomy[2]
vs.
open
laminectomy if
significant
bilateral disease

MIS
transpedicular
vertebrectomy
with
reconstruction[2]

Open posterior
laminectomy
with
stabilization

Open
posterolateral
or
anterior
approach

C

Thoracic vertebral
body fracture

Alignment well
preserved

Significant kyphotic
deformity/subluxation

Percutaneous pedicle
screw-rod
instrumentation ±
MIS decompression

Open decompression
and stabilization
with restoration of
alignment/fracture
reduction

[1]Minimally invasive thoracic microdiskectomy.
[2]Particularly suitable if limited life expectancy.

3

Posterior Thoracic Approaches for Disk Disease, Tumor, or Trauma

Frank L. Acosta Jr., David J. Moller, and John C. Liu

◆ Posterior Thoracic Approaches for Disk Disease

Disk herniation in the thoracic spine is a relatively uncommon phenomenon compared with the cervical or lumbar spine, and can be asymptomatic in up to 40% of cases.[1,2] When symptomatic, thoracic disk herniations can cause pain and/or neurological deficit and require surgical treatment.[3] Traditional surgical approaches for thoracic disk removal fall into three main categories: (1) posterior/posterolateral (laminectomy, transpedicular, costotransversectomy), (2) lateral (extracavitary), and (3) anterior (transthoracic). Although each can be successful in treating a symptomatic herniated thoracic disk, these traditional open surgical approaches require extensive dissection of the posterior paraspinous muscles (posterior and lateral approaches), significant removal of the bony elements of the thoracic spine (transpedicular) and associated ribs (costotransversectomy, extracavitary), or violation of the thoracic cavity (transthoracic) to access the thoracic disk space. As such, each of these traditional techniques can be associated with a significant amount of postoperative approach-related morbidity, including paraspinal muscle atrophy (posterior and lateral approaches), reduced ventilatory capacity (anterior approach), and increased postoperative pain (posterior, lateral, anterior approaches).[4–9]

The goal of any minimally invasive surgical technique is the reduction of approach-related morbidity. Minimally invasive spine surgery specifically causes less disruption of normal tissue and, in proficient hands, is associated with less operative blood loss and operative time, resulting in reduced postoperative morbidity, shorter hospital stays, and shorter recovery times compared with traditional open approaches.[1,10,11] Because the approach-related morbidity associated with traditional approaches to the thoracic disk space can be significant, minimally invasive surgical techniques can be particularly valuable in treating symptomatic herniated thoracic disks. While the traditional unilateral subperiosteal exposure for a transpedicular thoracic diskectomy can be performed with relative ease in the very thin patient, exposure in an obese patient requires a longer incision and greater muscular dissection with associated blood loss. The use of tubular retractors can be particularly useful in this patient population when considering the transpedicular or costotransversectomy approach. This section will describe a minimal-access posterior approach to the thoracic disk space, the minimally invasive thoracic microdiskectomy (MITM). This technique uses a posterolateral transforaminal/transfacet approach to the thoracic disk space and can be performed with the use of an endoscope or microscope,[1,12] depending upon the surgeon's experience.

Preoperative Evaluation

Although most often manifesting as thoracic radiculopathy, myelopathy, or back pain, thoracic disk herniations can present with a wide variety of symptoms, including shoulder or abdominal pain or angina-like symptoms,[13-15] and a thorough history and physical examination are therefore crucial to the accurate diagnosis of a symptomatic herniated thoracic disk. The preoperative radiographic evaluation of a suspected herniated thoracic disk should include magnetic resonance imaging (MRI) and/or postmyelogram computed tomography (CT). Although an MRI scan provides excellent anatomical and soft tissue detail, the CT/CT myelogram is helpful for assessing the degree of spinal cord compression and for delineating the extent of calcification of a herniated thoracic disk. Additionally, anteroposterior (AP) and lateral thoracic and lumbar plain radiographs should be ordered to assess the number of ribs and lumbar vertebrae to ensure correct-level surgery. A chest radiograph is helpful to determine the number of ribs for intraoperative localization. Because the localization of the correct thoracic level is difficult yet of utmost importance, at least two methods should be used for intraoperative localization to avoid wrong-level surgery.[12]

Soft central and lateral, as well as calcified lateral, thoracic disks are best suited for MITM (**Fig. 3.1**). For central calcified thoracic disks, we prefer to use an anterior thoracoscopic approach to ensure adequate cord decompression with minimal thecal sac manipulation.

Operative Technique

After induction of general endotracheal anesthesia, an arterial line, Foley catheter, and evoked potential (motor and somatosensory) electrodes are inserted. Although evoked potential monitoring is not required in every setting, we use it routinely at our institution. The patient is then positioned prone on a radiolucent Wilson frame with proper padding of all pressure points. The operative field is prepped and draped in the usual sterile fashion. A C-arm fluoroscope is then brought into the field in a sterile manner. The fluoroscope monitor is positioned opposite the surgeon, who is standing on the side ipsilateral to the disk herniation or the side of the most severe symptoms. AP fluoroscopic images are then taken to indicate the approximate location of the desired level, using a K-wire held on the end of a needle driver so that the surgeon's hand is

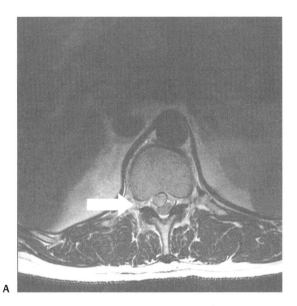

A

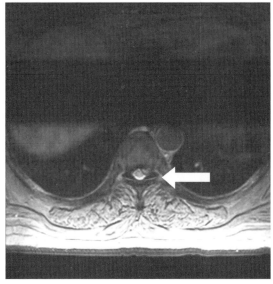

B

Fig. 3.1 **(A)** Preoperative magnetic resonance imaging showing noncalcified (soft) para-central and **(B)** lateral herniated thoracic disk with spinal cord compression (*white arrows*). These types of thoracic disk herniations would be amenable to minimally invasive thoracic microdiskectomy.

out of the field of view. The proper level is located by counting from the last rib up and from the first rib down and ensuring that these two methods are in agreement. It is important to note the number of ribs on preoperative chest and thoracic spine radiographs and correlate this with intraoperative localization. The location of the appropriate level is then marked on the skin with a skin marker and the C-arm is rotated to allow for lateral fluoroscopy. Lateral fluoroscopic images are then used to confirm the proper level by counting up from the sacrum. During this process, it is important to note the number of lumbar vertebrae seen on preoperative imaging. It is important to make sure that all methods used to confirm proper location are in agreement.

After proper localization, a skin incision (~2 cm long) is made, centered on the desired level, ~3 to 5 cm lateral to midline. The fascia is then incised sharply and a K-wire is inserted so as to come into contact with the transverse process of the caudal vertebra at the level of interest. This is confirmed using the C-arm. Care should be taken when passing the K-wire so as to avoid inserting the K-wire too deeply into the spinal canal or pleural space. After the K-wire is docked against the transverse process, the first muscle dilator is passed using C-arm guidance over the K-wire, and the K-wire is removed. Then a series of sequentially larger tubular muscle dilators are inserted over each other, followed by the placement of a tubular muscle retractor. The muscle retractor is attached to a flexible arm that is secured to the contralateral side of the operating table, and the dilators are then removed. The center of the tubular retractor should be positioned over the desired disk space on lateral fluoroscopic images. AP and lateral C-arm images are taken again at this point to confirm the proper level.

The microscope is then draped and brought into the field. Electrocautery is used to remove all overlying soft tissue and muscle so that the proximal aspect of the transverse process–facet junction is visualized. Next, a high-speed pneumatic drill is used to drill the cephalad aspect of the proximal transverse process of the inferior vertebra and lateral facet complex overlying the disk space. The pedicle of the caudal vertebra is then identified and traced back to the disk space, drilling the cephalad aspect of this pedicle as necessary to access the disk space. The lateral thecal sac is also visualized at this point. Radiographic confirmation of the disk space is obtained by placing a number 4 Penfield on the annulus and taking a lateral C-arm image.

The disk annulus and overlying epidural veins are then coagulated with bipolar electrocautery and the annulus is sharply incised with a #15 or #11 blade. Next, the diskectomy is performed with a combination of pituitary rongeurs, down-pushing curettes, and a Woodson elevator. Soft lateral disk herniations are removed under direct visualization. For soft central disk herniations, enough disk material should be removed to allow for delivery of the herniated fragment into the disk space using a down-pushing curette or a Woodson elevator. Calcified lateral disk herniations may require drilling of the rostral or caudal posterolateral vertebral body to allow for removal without manipulation of the thecal sac. Adequate decompression of the spinal cord and dura is ensured by inspecting the ventral epidural space with a Woodson elevator or similar instrument. Following completion of the diskectomy, adequate hemostasis is obtained and the thoracodorsal fascia closed with interrupted 0-Vicryl sutures (Ethicon Inc., Somerville, NJ), followed by interrupted 3–0 Vicryl sutures for the subdermal layer. Skin closure may be secured with either Steri-Strips (3M, St. Paul, MN) or a dermal adhesive.

◆ Posterior Thoracic Approaches for Tumor

Although the specific goals of surgical treatment of thoracic spinal tumors depend upon the tumor type and location, stage, comorbidities, life expectancy, and extent of spinal involvement, the general goals of neural element decompression, tumor resection, restoration of anatomical alignment, and stabilization in cases of spinal instability are usually a part of most surgical spinal oncologic treatment strategies. Because these goals have traditionally been accomplished via open surgical approaches to the thoracic spine, they have usually carried with them significant morbidity and complication rates for the patient with a thoracic spinal tumor.[16–18] Many spinal oncology patients have limited life expectancies from their underlying disease and greater comorbidities, and so minimizing perioperative morbidity is of utmost importance. As such, the application of minimally invasive surgical techniques has the potential to be of great benefit to patients with spinal tumors. Various studies have shown that minimally invasive techniques for thoracic spinal tumor resection result in reduced intensive care unit (ICU) stay, reduced perioperative morbidity and pain, expedited ambulation, and early hospital discharge compared with open techniques.[19,20]

Strategies for the minimally invasive surgical treatment of thoracic spinal tumors depend upon tumor location relative to a vertebral segment (i.e., involvement of anterior and/or posterior elements). For tumors involving the posterior column and causing neural element compromise, posterior decompression can be achieved via tubular hemilaminectomy. If significant bilateral disease exists dorsally, a standard open laminectomy approach is most appropriate. For tumors of the vertebral body, direct neural element decompression and tumor resection can be achieved via posterolateral minimally invasive transpedicular vertebrectomy. This approach must be weighed against the possibility of limited tumor resection and a less robust fixation from a more narrow exposure. Patients with a limited life expectancy would be appropriate candidates. Subsequent anterior column reconstruction can simultaneously be accomplished with this approach.[21] This section describes techniques for anterior and posterior column decompression of the thoracic spine in the setting of spinal tumors, as well as subsequent anterior column reconstruction and stabilization.

Preoperative Evaluation

Following a detailed history and physical examination, the preoperative radiographic evaluation should include a CT scan and MRI of the thoracic spine to define the bony (CT) and soft tissue (MRI) pathology of the tumor and adjacent segments. For metastatic disease, preoperative staging to define the extent of systemic tumor burden should be performed with a CT scan of the chest, abdomen, and pelvis. Postmyelographic CT is also useful to evaluate spinal canal compromise. As mentioned previously, plain lumbar and thoracic spine radiographs, as well as a chest x-ray, are important in the preoperative radiographic workup to assess number of ribs and lumbar vertebrae to ensure proper intraoperative localization.

Tumors involving the posterior elements and causing spinal cord compression are suitable for treatment via minimally invasive hemilaminectomy and decompression. Tumors affecting the vertebral body, encroaching upon the ventral spinal canal, can be resected and the thecal sac directly decompressed via a minimally invasive transpedicular vertebrectomy (with reconstruction).[21,22]

Operative Technique

Posterior Decompression (Hemilaminectomy)

After induction of general endotracheal anesthesia, a Foley catheter, arterial line, and evoked potential leads are inserted. The patient is then positioned prone on a radiolucent Wilson frame with proper padding of all pressure points. Using a combination of AP and lateral fluoroscopy, the proper level is identified and marked on the skin with a skin marker. The field is then prepped and draped in the usual sterile fashion.

A skin incision is made, ~2 cm long and centered on the desired level, ~3 to 5 cm lateral to midline on the side of the tumor (if eccentric) or the side of the most severe symptoms (if the tumor is midline). The fascia is then incised sharply and a K-wire is inserted so as to come into contact with the transverse process of the level of interest. This is confirmed using the C-arm. After the K-wire is docked against the transverse process, the first muscle dilator is passed using C-arm guidance over the K-wire and the K-wire removed. Then a series of sequentially larger tubular muscle dilators are inserted over each other, followed by the placement of a tubular muscle retractor. The muscle retractor is attached to a flexible arm that is secured to the contralateral side of the operating table, and the dilators are then removed. The center of the tubular retractor should be positioned over the lamina of the level of interest on lateral fluoroscopic images. AP and lateral C-arm images are taken again at this point to confirm the proper level.

The operating microscope is then brought into the field and draped. Electrocautery is used to remove all overlying soft tissue, and the tubular retractor is repositioned as necessary so that the junction of the lamina and spinous process is clearly visible. The angle of the tubular retractor at this point is usually directed ~20 degrees toward the midline. Once the bone anatomy is identified, a high-speed pneumatic drill is used to remove the ipsilateral lamina and tumor down to the ligamentum flavum. The laminectomy should be carried laterally to the level of the medial pedicle, taking care to preserve the pars interarticularis. After completion of the ipsilateral laminectomy, contralateral posterior spinal canal decompression and tumor resection are begun by undermining the spinous process with the high-speed drill. The tubular retractor is then repositioned to allow for visualization of the spinal canal across the midline, usually angled ~30 to 45 degrees from lateral to medial. The contralateral lamina is resected with the drill in an inside-out direction. Care should be taken to preserve the ligamentum flavum until bone resection is complete. Adequate contralateral canal decompression is confirmed by palpating the contralateral pedicle and neural foramina with a nerve hook or Woodson elevator.

Once the bony decompression and tumor resection have been completed, attention is turned to removal of the ligamentum flavum. The ligament may be incised sharply with a #15 blade or entered with a nerve hook to allow for insertion of a small curette or Kerrison rongeur. The ligament is then removed using these instruments, with repositioning of the tubular retractor as necessary, until the entire thecal sac and proximal nerve roots are visualized. Decompression of the spinal canal and neural foramen is then carefully checked with a fine probe. After posterior decompression and tumor resection are confirmed, the field is irrigated and hemostasis achieved. The fascia and skin are then closed in the usual fashion.

Anterior Column Decompression (Transpedicular Vertebrectomy)

Endotracheal anesthesia is induced, and monitoring, positioning, and localization are performed as previously described. A 2.5 to 3 cm long skin incision is made 2 cm lateral to the midline (6 cm lateral to the midline if an extracavitary vertebrectomy is to be performed) on the more involved side and carried through the thoracodorsal fascia. Blunt finger dissection is then used to palpate the transverse process and proximal rib. An expandable tubular muscle retractor (METRx Quadrant retractor system, Medtronic, Memphis, TN) is then inserted over tubular dilators in the usual manner and angled ~30 degrees toward the midline (**Fig. 3.2A**).

The operating microscope is then brought into the field and draped. Electrocautery is used to remove all overlying soft tissue. The transverse process, lamina, and thoracic pedicle are then removed with a high-speed drill (**Fig. 3.2B**). The ligamentum flavum is removed to allow for visualization of the lateral thecal sac and exiting nerve root. The thoracic nerve root can be transected at this point, if necessary, to allow for improved visualization of the ventrolateral thoracic spinal canal and posterior vertebral body. The high-speed drill and curettes are then used to perform the vertebrectomy and tumor resection. Pituitary rongeurs can also be used to remove soft tumor in a piecemeal fashion. Ventral epidural tumor can be delivered into the vertebrectomy defect with down-pushing curettes or down-biting pituitary rongeurs. Because of the posterolateral trajectory of the tubular retractor, the lateral 25% of the ventral spinal canal can be directly visualized and decompressed, and indirect decompression can be accomplished over 75% of the ventral surface (**Fig. 3.2C**).[22] A bilateral approach can facilitate complete decompression of the ventral spinal canal

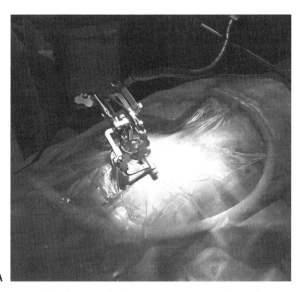

A

Fig. 3.2 **(A)** Photograph of operative setup with Quadrant retractor (Medtronic, Memphis, TN) in place to perform minimally invasive thoracic transpedicular vertebrectomy in a cadaver. (*continued*)

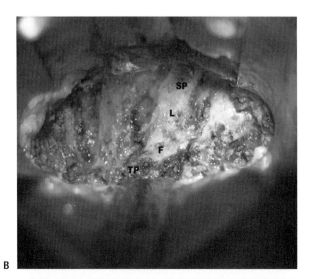

B

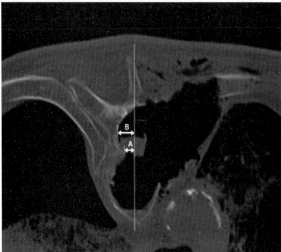

C

Fig. 3.2 (*continued*)   **(B)** Photograph showing visualization of the spinous process (SP), lamina (L), facet (F) and transverse process (TP) through the expandable retractor after removal of the overlying soft tissue. **(C)** Postprocedural computed tomographic scan after minimally invasive transpedicular thoracic vertebrectomy from a left-sided approach in a cadaver. Note that almost the entire ventral and dorsal thecal sac can be decompressed from a unilateral approach. Shown are the decompressed contralateral spinal canal (*arrow* A) and half of the interpedicular distance (*arrow* B).

and thecal sac, though subsequent instrumentation is required after bilateral trans-pedicular approaches. Complete decompression is ensured by passing a Woodson elevator or similar instrument into the ventral epidural space.

Following vertebrectomy, reconstruction of the anterior column is performed with an appropriately sized expandable titanium cage.[21] The cage is inserted into the vertebrectomy defect and expanded until secure. Following appropriate stabilization, the skin and fascia are closed in the usual fashion. Posterior column fixation can then be performed, as necessary, in the same position. Posterior pedicle screw–rod instrumentation is described in the next section.

◆ Posterior Thoracic Approaches for Trauma

The basic tenets of the surgical treatment of spinal trauma include decompression of the neural elements, reduction and realignment of dislocated vertebral segments, and stabilization via anterior and/or posterior column instrumentation and fusion. These goals have traditionally been accomplished using standard open approaches to the thoracic spine. Patients with spinal trauma, however, have been reported to be at risk for increased operative blood loss and infection.[21,23] Therefore, reducing perioperative morbidity with the application of minimally invasive surgical approaches to treat spinal trauma has the potential to be especially beneficial for this patient population.[24] The principles and techniques of minimally invasive posterior approaches for circumferential thoracic spinal canal decompression were described in the previous section. Posterior percutaneous pedicle screw–rod fixation for stabilization of thoracic spinal fractures has been reported by several groups[24–26] and has been found to significantly reduce blood loss while maintaining the same amount of correction and fixation as with open techniques.[25] Percutaneous fixation techniques for traumatic fractures are most appropriate in the absence of significant malalignment or neural element compromise.

Preoperative Evaluation

Thoracic spinal fractures are usually noted initially on plain AP and lateral chest radiographs, or dedicated AP and lateral plain films of the thoracic spine. Detailed bony anatomy of the spinal fracture is best visualized on a CT scan, with sagittal and coronal reconstructions. Vertebral body height loss, fracture pattern, fracture fragments, angulation, and subluxation are best visualized on CT scans. MRI should also be obtained and is useful for detecting soft tissue abnormalities, such as hematomas, traumatic thoracic disk herniations, and ligamentous injury.

Operative Technique

After induction of general endotracheal anesthesia, an arterial line, Foley catheter, and evoked potential (motor and somatosensory) electrodes are inserted. The patient is then positioned prone on a radiolucent Wilson frame. The C-arm is then brought into the field and used to localize the appropriate levels to be instrumented. Again, proper localization is often difficult, yet of utmost importance, in the thoracic spine. The appropriate levels should be marked on the skin. The pedicles of all levels to be instrumented must be visualized on C-arm fluoroscopy in order for percutaneous instrumentation to be performed (**Fig. 3.3A**). The use of two C-arms (one in the lateral and one in the AP position) can facilitate the procedure. Proper alignment of the C-arm is crucial to obtaining true AP and lateral views of the thoracic vertebral body and pedicles. In a true AP image, both the anterior and posterior superior end plates line up to produce a single end plate. In addition, the pedicles should appear just below the superior end plate, and the spinous process should be in the midline between the pedicles. A true lateral image also demonstrates a single end plate, superimposed pedicles, and a single posterior vertebral body wall shadow (ensuring absence of rotation).[27]

Following appropriate localization, the surgical field is prepped and draped in the usual sterile fashion. The skin incision is marked ~1 cm lateral to the lateral wall of the pedicle to allow for a medial-to-lateral trajectory of screw insertion. A 1 cm incision is then made through the skin and fascia, a Jamshidi needle is then carefully inserted and docked against the bone, and an AP C-arm image is obtained. The Jamshidi needle is then repositioned as necessary to lie directly over the lateral wall of the pedicle. The Jamshidi needle is then gently malleted to penetrate the posterior cortical bone, and another AP image is obtained to ensure proper needle trajectory. With the proper trajectory, the needle is then again malleted to pass into and down the pedicle. Serial AP and lateral fluoroscopic images are taken to monitor the progress of the needle and ensure that the proper trajectory is maintained. When the tip of the needle reaches the posterior vertebral body cortex on the lateral image, the needle tip should be no more than halfway (from lateral to medial) across the pedicle on an AP image. The needle is passed just beyond the posterior vertebral body wall into the vertebral body, and the stylet is then removed, allowing for insertion of a K-wire. Soft, cancellous bone within the vertebral body should be palpable with a K-wire. After removal of the Jamshidi needle over the K-wire, a lateral C-arm image should be taken to ensure that the K-wire is appropriately positioned approximately midway through the vertebral body. It is important to secure and monitor the K-wire until removal to ensure that it does not migrate anteriorly and penetrate the anterior vertebral body cortex. All pedicles to be instrumented are cannulated in a similar fashion and attention is turned to pedicle preparation and screw insertion (**Fig. 3.3B**).

Following proper K-wire placement, an appropriately sized cannulated tap is then inserted over the K-wire and used to tap the pedicle. Again, the K-wire should be secured at all times, and lateral fluoroscopic images should be serially taken during tapping to ensure that the K-wire does not migrate. After tapping, an appropriately sized pedicle screw with screw extension is then inserted over the K-wire in a similar fashion (**Fig. 3.3C**). Once the pedicle screw is approximately midway through the pedicle, the K-wire can be removed and the pedicle screw advanced until secure. After all screws have been placed, a rod is introduced into the screw heads, and set screws are used to secure the rod (**Fig. 3.3C**). Compression or distraction can be performed, as necessary, prior to final tightening of the set screws. After final tightening, the screw extensions are removed and the fascia closed in the usual manner (**Fig. 3.3D**).

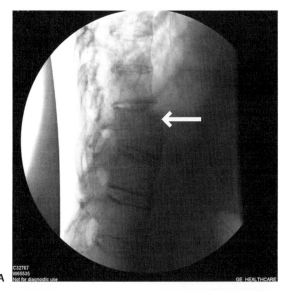

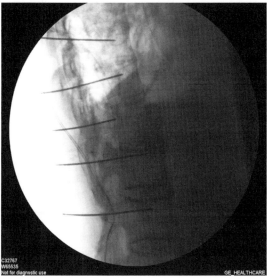

Fig. 3.3 **(A)** Intraoperative lateral fluoroscopic image of an 87-year-old woman with severe back pain after a fall at home demonstrating a T7 fracture-dislocation (*arrow*) requiring internal pedicle screw–rod bracing. **(B)** Lateral C-arm image after K-wire cannulation of pedicles from T5 to T9. (*continued*)

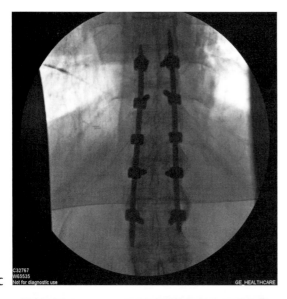

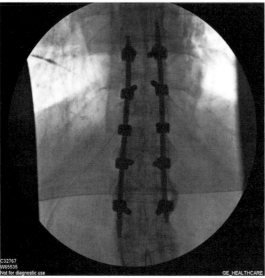

Fig. 3.3 (*continued*)   **(C)** Lateral fluoroscopy after pedicle screw placement over K-wires demonstrating pedicle screw extensions and showing insertion of the connecting rod (Longitude, Medtronic, Memphis, TN). **(D)** Intraoperative anteroposterior fluoroscopic image demonstrating bilateral pedicle screw–rod fixation from T5 to T9.

◆ Conclusions

Traditional, open surgical approaches to the thoracic spine are associated with significant perioperative morbidity. Minimally invasive posterior approaches to the thoracic spine have been associated with decreased blood loss, operative time, postoperative morbidity, and hospitalization time. These approaches have been applied to the treatment of various pathologies of the thoracic spine, including herniated thoracic disks (transfacet approach), tumors of the posterior (hemilaminectomy approach) and anterior columns (transpedicular vertebrectomy), and thoracic spinal fracture (percutaneous approach for pedicle screw–rod insertion). Proper localization is probably the most important step in the surgical treatment of thoracic spinal pathologies. As these minimally invasive techniques continue to be applied and new ones are developed, it is important for spinal surgeons to continue to assess their impact on patient outcomes and compare these outcomes to those of patients treated with traditional open techniques.

References

1. Perez-Cruet MJ, Kim BS, Sandhu F, Samartzis D, Fessler RG. Thoracic microendoscopic discectomy. J Neurosurg Spine 2004;1:58–63
2. Brown CW, Deffer PA Jr, Akmakjian J, Donaldson DH, Brugman JL. The natural history of thoracic disc herniation. Spine (Phila Pa 1976) 1992;17(6, Suppl):S97–S102
3. Lidar Z, Lifshutz J, Bhattacharjee S, Kurpad SN, Maiman DJ. Minimally invasive, extracavitary approach for thoracic disc herniation: technical report and preliminary results. Spine J 2006;6:157–163
4. Faciszewski T, Winter RB, Lonstein JE, Denis F, Johnson L. The surgical and medical perioperative complications of anterior spinal fusion surgery in the thoracic and lumbar spine in adults: a review of 1223 procedures. Spine (Phila Pa 1976) 1995;20:1592–1599
5. Weber BR, Grob D, Dvořák J, Müntener M. Posterior surgical approach to the lumbar spine and its effect on the multifidus muscle. Spine (Phila Pa 1976) 1997;22:1765–1772
6. Rantanen J, Hurme M, Falck B, et al. The lumbar multifidus muscle five years after surgery for a lumbar intervertebral disc herniation. Spine (Phila Pa 1976) 1993;18:568–574
7. Kim DY, Lee SH, Chung SK, Lee HY. Comparison of multifidus muscle atrophy and trunk extension muscle strength: percutaneous versus open pedicle screw fixation. Spine (Phila Pa 1976) 2005;30:123–129
8. Jackson RK. The long-term effects of wide laminectomy for lumbar disc excision. A review of 130 patients. J Bone Joint Surg Br 1971;53:609–616
9. McDonnell MF, Glassman SD, Dimar JR II, Puno RM, Johnson JR. Perioperative complications of anterior procedures on the spine. J Bone Joint Surg Am 1996;78:839–847
10. Perez-Cruet MJ, Fessler RG, Perin NI. Review: complications of minimally invasive spinal surgery. Neurosurgery 2002;51(5, Suppl):S26–S36
11. Perez-Cruet MJ, Foley KT, Isaacs RE, et al. Microendoscopic lumbar discectomy: technical note. Neurosurgery 2002;51(5, Suppl):S129–S136
12. Sheikh H, Samartzis D, Perez-Cruet MJ. Techniques for the operative management of thoracic disc herniation: minimally invasive thoracic microdiscectomy. Orthop Clin North Am 2007;38:351–361, abstract vi
13. Wilke A, Wolf U, Lageard P, Griss P. Thoracic disc herniation: a diagnostic challenge. Man Ther 2000;5:181–184
14. Rohde RS, Kang JD. Thoracic disc herniation presenting with chronic nausea and abdominal pain: a case report. J Bone Joint Surg Am 2004;86-A:379–381

15. Eleraky MA, Apostolides PJ, Dickman CA, Sonntag VK. Herniated thoracic discs mimic cardiac disease: three case reports. Acta Neurochir (Wien) 1998;140:643–646

16. Vitaz TW, Oishi M, Welch WC, Gerszten PC, Disa JJ, Bilsky MH. Rotational and transpositional flaps for the treatment of spinal wound dehiscence and infections in patient populations with degenerative and oncological disease. J Neurosurg 2004;100(1, Suppl Spine):46–51

17. Wang JC, Boland P, Mitra N, et al. Single-stage posterolateral transpedicular approach for resection of epidural metastatic spine tumors involving the vertebral body with circumferential reconstruction: results in 140 patients. Invited submission from the Joint Section Meeting on Disorders of the Spine and Peripheral Nerves, March 2004. J Neurosurg Spine 2004;1:287–298

18. North RB, LaRocca VR, Schwartz J, et al. Surgical management of spinal metastases: analysis of prognostic factors during a 10-year experience. J Neurosurg Spine 2005;2:564–573

19. Huang TJ, Hsu RW, Li YY, Cheng CC. Minimal access spinal surgery (MASS) in treating thoracic spine metastasis. Spine (Phila Pa 1976) 2006;31:1860–1863

20. Scheufler KM. Technique and clinical results of minimally invasive reconstruction and stabilization of the thoracic and thoracolumbar spine with expandable cages and ventrolateral plate fixation. Neurosurgery 2007;61:798–808

21. Smith JS, Ogden AT, Fessler RG. Minimally invasive posterior thoracic fusion. Neurosurg Focus 2008;25:E9

22. Deutsch H, Boco T, Lobel J. Minimally invasive transpedicular vertebrectomy for metastatic disease to the thoracic spine. J Spinal Disord Tech 2008;21:101–105

23. Verlaan JJ, Diekerhof CH, Buskens E, et al. Surgical treatment of traumatic fractures of the thoracic and lumbar spine: a systematic review of the literature on techniques, complications, and outcome. Spine (Phila Pa 1976) 2004;29:803–814

24. Rampersaud YR, Annand N, Dekutoski MB. Use of minimally invasive surgical techniques in the management of thoracolumbar trauma: current concepts. Spine (Phila Pa 1976) 2006;31(11, Suppl):S96–S102

25. Wild MH, Glees M, Plieschnegger C, Wenda K. Five-year follow-up examination after purely minimally invasive posterior stabilization of thoracolumbar fractures: a comparison of minimally invasive percutaneously and conventionally open treated patients. Arch Orthop Trauma Surg 2007;127:335–343

26. Ringel F, Stoffel M, Stüer C, Meyer B. Minimally invasive transmuscular pedicle screw fixation of the thoracic and lumbar spine. Neurosurgery 2006;59(4, Suppl 2):ONS361–ONS366

27. Anderson DG, Samartzis D, Shen FH, Tannoury C. Percutaneous instrumentation of the thoracic and lumbar spine. Orthop Clin North Am 2007;38:401–408, abstract vii

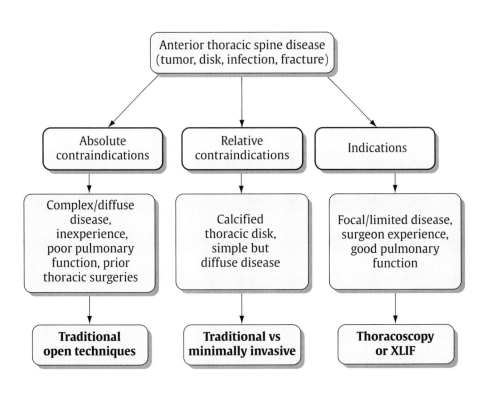

4

Anterior Thoracic Approaches for Disk Disease, Tumor, or Trauma

Isaac O. Karikari and Robert E. Isaacs

The anterior vertebral body of the cervicothoracic and thoracic spine houses the vast majority of pathological processes. The initial impetus for development of anterior surgical approaches stemmed from tuberculous involvement of the thoracic spine.[1] Although the incidence of spinal tuberculosis has decreased, the thoracic spine is nevertheless commonly accessed for a variety of pathological processes. This includes degenerative, infectious, traumatic, neoplastic, and congenital diseases. The development of minimally invasive techniques has expanded the feasibility of accessing virtually all parts of the thoracic spine that are normally accessed via open techniques through smaller incisions. The anterior upper thoracic spine (T1–4) still remains a relatively inaccessible area to both open and minimally invasive techniques due to the sternoclavicular joint, manubrium, and neurovascular structures. The minimally invasive surgical techniques to the anterior thoracic spine have emerged from modifications of the traditional open techniques. Thoracoscopic and the extreme lateral interbody fusion are now the two primary minimally invasive approaches to the anterior thoracic spine.

◆ Thoracoscopic Approaches

Mack et al were the first to report the application of thoracoscopy to treatment of thoracic spinal diseases.[2] Through lessons learned from their in vivo porcine models, thoracoscopic instruments for spine surgery were developed and utilized initially for tissue biopsy and drainage of vertebral abscesses. Their work, however, was preceded by years of gradual application of endoscopic techniques to the lumbar spine such

Table 4.1   Indications for Thoracoscopic Spine Surgery

Degenerative	Trauma	Infection	Deformity	Tumor	Other
Herniated disk	Fracture stabilization and fixation	Debridement Biopsy	Anterior release for scoliosis and Scheuermann kyphosis	Primary and metastatic tumor resections Biopsy	Sympathectomy Thoracoplasty

as the use of the myeloscope to perform disk space biopsies in 1946.[3] Thoracoscopic spine surgery has now become an established entity of minimally invasive surgery, with several groups reporting excellent outcomes.[4,5]

Indications and Contraindications

In general, the indications for thoracoscopic spine surgery are the same as the traditional open techniques. The indications are listed in **Table 4.1**. Thoracic sympathectomies, followed by diskectomies, appear to be the most commonly performed thoracoscopic procedures. In a retrospective review of 241 thoracoscopic procedures reported by Han et al, there were 164 sympathectomies, 60 diskectomies, five neurogenic tumor resections, eight corpectomies for spinal reconstructions, two anterior releases, and two biopsies.[4]

Thoracoscopic spine surgery is contraindicated in patients with severe respiratory insufficiency, high airway pressures, patients with previous multiple anterior thoracic procedures with subsequent scarring and adhesions, and inability to tolerate single-lung ventilation.

Thoracoscopic Spine Technique

Operating Room Setup and Patient Positioning

The operating room is set up in a standard fashion, similar to that for any thoracoscopic surgery and allowing the patient to be placed into either a Trendelenburg, reverse Trendelenburg, anterior, or posterior position. The operating table must be radiolucent to allow fluoroscopic imaging. After double-lumen intubation, the patient is placed in a lateral decubitus position. Although most surgeons prefer a right-sided approach, the anatomy of the aorta and azygous veins ultimately determines the side of approach. All necessary pressure points should be adequately padded. For high thoracic approaches, the shoulders should be flexed more than 90 degrees, and the axilla should be prepped and draped. The iliac crest is prepped in cases where bone grafting is anticipated. The spine surgeon and first assistant (usually a thoracic surgeon) stand on the abdominal side (ventral) of the patient and face one monitor. A third assistant stands on the dorsal aspect of the patient and faces the second monitor. The operating room nurse stands to the right or left of the third assistant.

Equipment

Although the instruments used in each thoracoscopic surgery differ by surgeon choice and surgical indication, the standard equipment used for most thoracoscopic spine surgery includes a 30 degree endoscope (10 mm in diameter for adults and 5 mm for children), fan lung retractor, harmonic scalpel, long-tipped electrocautery device, Cobb elevators, curettes, pituitary/Kerrison rongeurs, suction-irrigation devices, and an endoscopic high-speed burr. Three to four trocars, 10 to 12 mm in diameter and 50 mm in length, are used to access the thoracic cavity.

Surgical Technique

The vertebral levels to be operated on are carefully identified with fluoroscopic guidance, and the disk space and anterior and posterior margins of the vertebral body are marked on the patient's skin. A 1 to 2 cm incision is made at the sixth, seventh, or eighth intercostal space along the medial axillary line for the first port for the thoracoscope. An exploratory thoracoscopy is then performed to expose the pleura and verify collapse of the ipsilateral lung. The remaining trocars are placed three intercostal spaces above or below the first trocar based on the location of the pathology. The next step is dependent on the surgical indication and will be described separately.

Thoracoscopic Surgery for Herniated Disk

Following radiographic confirmation of the appropriate level, the patient is approached on the side of the herniated disk. For central herniated disks (**Fig. 4.1**), the patient is typically approached from the right side. The trocars are then placed under direct visualization. The lungs are then retracted using a fan retractor. The proximal 2 to 3 cm of the rib head is removed with a high-speed burr, osteotome, or pituitary rongeur for all cases above T11 due to the insertion of the rib head below the disk space at this level. The rib head is disarticulated by releasing the costotransverse and costovertebral ligaments. Using a diamond burr and Kerrison rongeur, a small part of the superior part of the pedicle is removed to gain access to the spinal canal. A defect is then created ventral to the spinal canal. Under direct visualization, the herniated disk is removed with an angled curette using a sweeping motion away from the dura. A Penfield probe is placed in the disk space followed by a fluoroscopic image to determine the extent of the decompression. A 24 French chest tube is typically inserted prior to reexpansion of lung and wound closure.

Thoracoscopic Surgery for Spinal Deformity

Anterior release for scoliosis and kyphosis can be performed adequately through endoscopic techniques.[6] The technique begins with exploratory thoracoscopy to remove all soft tissues. The pleura overlying the apex of the scoliosis curve is incised in a longitudinal fashion. A diskectomy or multilevel diskectomies are next performed meticulously without interrupting the blood supply to the spinal cord via the segmental vessels. The azygous vein is identified and protected before releasing the anterior longitudinal ligament of the concave side of the curve using a Kerrison rongeur. After adequate hemostasis, a 24 French chest tube is placed prior to wound closure.

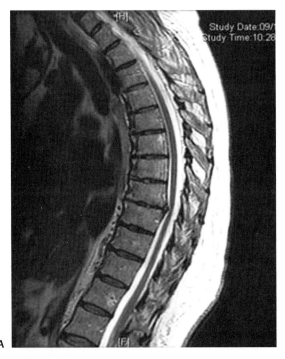

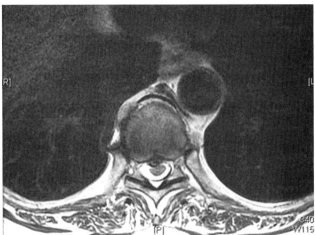

Fig. 4.1   (A) Sagittal and **(B)** axial T2-weighted images of a T8–9 central disk removed via thoracoscopic approach. (*continued*)

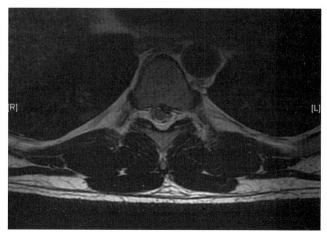

C

Fig. 4.1 (*continued*)   (**C**) Axial T2 image of a paracentral disk herniation less well suited for thoracoscopic approach due to location of aorta and azygous vein. This disk was removed with a posterolateral approach.

Thoracoscopic Surgical Technique for Fracture

Thoracic and thoracolumbar fractures can be adequately treated with thoracoscopic approaches with good outcomes.[7] In contrast to patients with herniated disks and spinal deformities, patients being treated for fractures tend to have associated injuries. As such, all necessary efforts are required to ensure medical stabilization prior to surgery.

After proper patient positioning as described earlier, the level of fracture and adjacent intact vertebral bodies are localized under fluoroscopic guidance. A 10 mm working channel is then centered over the site of the fracture. A right-sided approach is preferred for fractures between T4 and T8, whereas a left-sided approach is preferred for fractures between T9 and L2 to aid in mobilization of the diaphragm. Four trocars are inserted sequentially in the standard fashion. Using a closed fan-shaped retractor through a working port, the fracture area is exposed and confirmed by fluoroscopy. The closed fan retractor blades are then opened to retract the collapsed lung. Fracture reconstruction is then performed using any of the commercially available systems, such as the MACS-TL (B. Braun Medical Inc., Bethlehem, PA) or Z-Plate instrumentation set (Medtronic, Sofamor Daneck, Inc., Memphis, TN). Lateral and anteroposterior x-rays are obtained intraoperatively prior to extubation.

◆ The eXtreme Lateral Interbody Fusion

The eXtreme Lateral Interbody Fusion (XLIF, NuVasive, Inc., San Diego, CA) approach offers a minimally invasive approach to the anterior thoracic spine. The procedure is 90 degrees off midline or a true lateral approach and can be used to treat a variety of spinal disorders, such as degenerative, scoliotic, traumatic, infectious, and neoplastic diseases (**Fig. 4.2**).

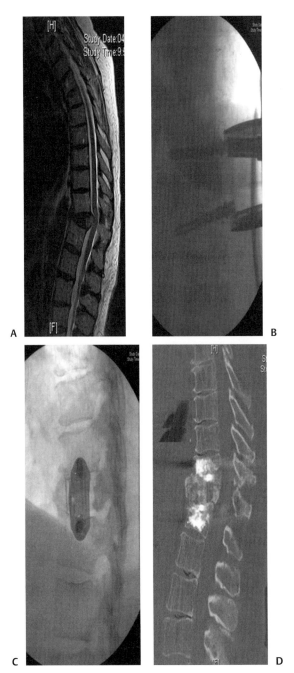

Fig. 4.2 Case illustration for a thoracic XLIF procedure. **(A)** Sagittal T2-weighted magnetic resonance imaging showing a T11 pathological fracture by tumor with canal compromise and subsequent kyphotic deformity. **(B)** Intraoperative x-ray showing T11 vertebrectomy with placement of an interbody cage and screw placement of T10 and T12. **(C)** Lateral x-ray showing restoration of vertebral column height. **(D)** Postoperative computed tomography at 1 year reveals solid fusion and maintenance of deformity correction.

As the lung is typically not deflated, standard single-lumen endotracheal intubation is performed. After endotracheal intubation, the patient is placed in a lateral position with all pressure points well padded. Prior to prepping and draping the patient, a true lateral film is obtained with fluoroscopy. Care is taken to ensure that the disk spaces/vertebrae are at a true 90 degree orientation to the floor. The corresponding vertebral bodies or disk spaces to be operated on are then marked on the patient's skin. The patient is prepped and draped in the sterile fashion. A 2 to 2.5 cm incision is made directly above the intended vertebral body level. After the incision, the patient is made apneic for a few seconds while a very small thoracotomy is made directly above the intended vertebral level, creating a pneumothorax. The surgeon's finger sweeps away the lung to protect it from injury, and a dilator (typically the second) is placed directly above the vertebral body. With the dilator safely positioned, a confirmatory x-ray is obtained and the necessary adjustments made to ensure proper positioning for the working channel. Using sequential dilations, a working channel is placed. It is imperative to provide intermittent ventilation during the positioning of dilators. At this time, a retractor system is positioned to avoid the lungs in the operative field. Full ventilatory support is resumed thereafter except in few instances when the retractor needs to be adjusted.

After adequate exposure is obtained, a diskectomy is performed in the standard fashion. If a corpectomy is planned, segmental arteries must be sacrificed. The vertebral body is gradually removed with the combination of a power drill, Kerrison rongeurs, and curettes creating a large defect ventral to the spinal canal proceeding from an anterior to posterior direction. Care must be taken to avoid violating the spinal canal. Once the vertebrectomy and associated diskectomies are completed, the posterior longitudinal ligament (PLL) is then removed to achieve a complete decompression. The placement of the prosthetic device then proceeds in a standard fashion. An in situ expandable spacer is advantageous given the limited space available. An anterior or posterior screw–rod construct is then considered. Periodic anterior posterior and lateral x-rays are taken during the vertebrectomy to ensure accurate positioning of the instrumentation. For simple and even multilevel diskectomies, the iatrogenic pneumothorax created in the initial stages of the procedure is decompressed and the chest tube removed in the recovery room after confirmatory x-ray of adequate decompression of the pneumothorax. The wound is then irrigated and closed in successive layers.

◆ Discussion

The advent of minimally invasive approaches to anterior thoracic spine diseases has provided a greater array of therapeutic options to treat these challenging conditions. Although video-assisted thoracoscopic techniques were initially used exclusively for simple diskectomies and soft tissue releases, their applications have been expanded now to include management of complex fractures, deformities, tumors, and degenerative diseases. Video-assisted spine surgery offers several significant advantages over traditional open approaches.

Some of the advantages of minimally invasive approaches to the thoracic spine include (1) minimal incisions; (2) decreased trauma to the chest wall resulting in less blood loss, fewer infections, less postoperative pain, improved respiratory function from less atelectasis, and shorter hospital stay[8,9]; and (3) improved visualization with a magnified 30 degree endoscope.

Despite the aforementioned advantages, there are drawbacks that need to be considered when contemplating a minimally invasive approach. The relative novelty of these approaches presents a significant learning curve to the surgeon and members of the operating team. This steep learning curve can therefore present several challenges to the inexperienced spine surgeon, leading to unexpected complications and longer operating times. It is advisable to attend several practical cadaver workshops and have a thoracic surgeon available to provide assistance as needed. For thoracoscopic procedures, the need for double-lumen, single-lung ventilation also presents challenges to the anesthesiologist.

◆ Conclusion

Several factors play a role in influencing the decision to use a thoracoscopic approach versus the XLIF approach. The greater the canal disease, the more one would favor thoracoscopic assistance. Although a hard calcified disk may be removed using either thoracoscopy or XLIF, a thoracoscopic approach will provide better visualization and triangulation of the pathology within the canal. The XLIF approach may be advantageous in a patient with poorer pulmonary mechanics given that no ipsilateral lung collapse is required. A thoracoscopic approach is best suited for multilevel instrumentation and compression techniques. Finally, and more importantly, surgeon comfort and familiarity with these techniques are perhaps the most influential factors when deciding between a thoracoscopic approach and the XLIF.

The aforementioned advantages of minimally invasive spine approaches to anterior thoracic spine diseases thus provide an excellent alternative to patients who cannot tolerate the traditional open surgery. Although the learning curve is daunting, once mastered, virtually any anterior thoracic disease can be treated successfully with minimal access in carefully selected patients.

References

1. Hodgson AR, Stock FE, Fang HS, Ong GB. Anterior spinal fusion: the operative approach and pathological findings in 412 patients with Pott's disease of the spine. Br J Surg 1960;48:172–178
2. Mack MJ, Regan JJ, Bobechko WP, Acuff TE. Application of thoracoscopy for diseases of the spine. Ann Thorac Surg 1993;56:736–738
3. Lindblom K. Diagnostic puncture of intervertebral disks in sciatica. Acta Orthop Scand 1948;17: 231–239
4. Han PP, Kenny K, Dickman CA. Thoracoscopic approaches to the thoracic spine: experience with 241 surgical procedures. Neurosurgery 2002;51(5, Suppl):S88–S95
5. Beisse R, Mückley T, Schmidt MH, Hauschild M, Bühren V. Surgical technique and results of endoscopic anterior spinal canal decompression. J Neurosurg Spine 2005;2:128–136

6. Regan JJ, Mack MJ, Picetti GD III. A technical report on video-assisted thoracoscopy in thoracic spinal surgery: preliminary description. Spine (Phila Pa 1976) 1995;20:831–837

7. Khoo LT, Beisse R, Potulski M. Thoracoscopic-assisted treatment of thoracic and lumbar fractures: a series of 371 consecutive cases. Neurosurgery 2002;51(5, Suppl):S104–S117

8. Ferson PF, Landreneau RJ, Dowling RD, et al. Comparison of open versus thoracoscopic lung biopsy for diffuse infiltrative pulmonary disease. J Thorac Cardiovasc Surg 1993;106:194–199

9. Landreneau RJ, Hazelrigg SR, Mack MJ, et al. Postoperative pain-related morbidity: video-assisted thoracic surgery versus thoracotomy. Ann Thorac Surg 1993;56:1285–1289

Section III

Lumbar Spine

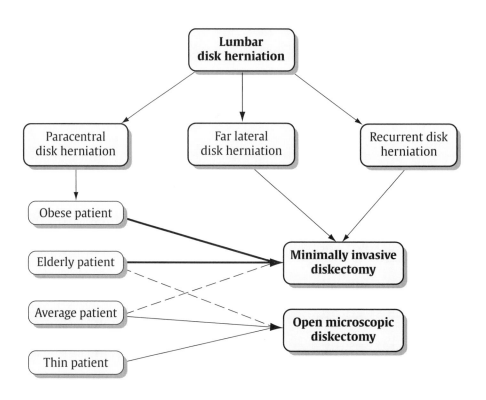

5

Minimally Invasive Lumbar Diskectomy

Amanda Muhs Saratsis, Faheem A. Sandhu, and Jean-Marc Voyadzis

Lumbar disk herniation causing radiculopathy from nerve root compression is one of the most common clinical problems managed by spine surgeons. Conservative management, consisting of judicious use of nonsteroidal antiinflammatory medications, limited bed rest, and in some cases physical therapy, lidocaine, or steroid injections, provides relief in the majority of cases. Patients with progressive neurological deficit or severe pain refractory to up to 6 weeks of conservative treatment warrant evaluation for surgical intervention.

Surgical options for the treatment of lumbar disk herniation include traditional open lumbar diskectomy involving subperiosteal dissection of the paraspinous muscles and retraction with a Taylor or Markham/Meyerding retractor, open lumbar microdiskectomy employing an operating microscope and Williams retractor, and minimally invasive microdiskectomy using a muscle-splitting approach and tubular retractors. The traditional approach for lumbar microdiskectomy and nerve root decompression has proven successful for short-term symptomatic relief of radicular leg pain in the majority of patients. When compared with a traditional approach to diskectomy, use of the operating microscope provides better anatomical visualization via a smaller skin incision to minimize potential complications, which include bleeding, infection, instability of the lumbar spine, persistent back pain and/or radicular pain, nerve root injury, dural tear, air embolism, injury to abdominal viscera, and/or major vascular injury.[1,2]

Refinement of the microsurgical approach has led to the development of minimally invasive techniques that utilize muscle-splitting tubular dilators aimed to minimize approach-related complications. Compared with an open microdiskectomy, a muscle-splitting, percutaneous approach to the lumbar disk space decreases the length of incision, minimizes soft tissue dissection by preserving natural tissue planes, and provides excellent visualization of the surgical anatomy. The demonstrated benefits include decreased postoperative pain, reduced length of hospital stay, and earlier mobilization and return to work, especially in patients with significant comorbidities.[3-5] The use of a minimally invasive approach for lumbar diskectomy is ideal for patients in whom the requisite larger incision and muscle dissection of an open approach could bring significant additional morbidity and make visualization of the surgical anatomy more challenging. In our opinion, this makes minimally invasive microdiskectomy the preferred approach over open microdiskectomy in elderly patients and in patients with far lateral disk herniation, recurrent disk disease, excessive soft tissue or paraspinal muscle atrophy, obesity, and multiple medical comorbidities. In contrast, for thin, young, healthy patients, the advantage of minimally invasive microdiskectomy compared with open microdiskectomy is debatable. Although the decision of surgical approach is usually dictated by surgeon experience and comfort level, certain pathologies and situations may be best treated using one technique as opposed to another. Increasing a surgeon's technique repertoire will greatly aid that surgeon in performing the best surgery for a given problem, rather than treating all problems with a single surgical technique.

◆ Preoperative Evaluation

All patients presenting with a history of leg pain suggestive of nerve root compression from disk herniation should undergo a detailed history and physical examination to ensure the pain is radicular in nature, to detect any motor or sensory deficit, and to rule out nonneurogenic etiologies for their pain. Imaging studies must be performed and should correlate the level of radiographic findings to the distribution of physical findings. Preoperative radiographic evaluation should include magnetic resonance imaging (MRI) or computed tomography (CT) myelogram to identify nerve root impingement secondary to disk herniation and detect the presence or absence of stenosis. In addition, anteroposterior (AP), lateral, and flexion-extension lumbar radiographs should be obtained to evaluate for the presence of instability. Patients most likely to benefit from surgical treatment are those presenting with unilateral radiculopathy who are without spinal instability or significant back pain, and who have failed 6 to 8 weeks of conservative management.

◆ Operative Technique

The patient is brought to the operating room where general endotracheal anesthesia is induced. The patient is placed prone on a Jackson table using a Wilson frame. The fluoroscopic monitor is placed at the foot of the patient opposite the operating surgeon for comfortable viewing. It is preferable to position the operating microscope base on the same side as the surgeon and the C-arm base on the opposite side. Should an endoscope be used, the viewing tower for endoscopic imaging is placed opposite to the surgeon with the C-arm base on the same side.

After the patient is positioned, a preoperative localizing radiograph is obtained with a Steinmann pin using lateral fluoroscopy to determine the operative level and plan the surgical approach. Once the appropriate disk level(s) is(are) identified, the site of entry is marked 1.5 cm lateral to midline, ipsilateral to the pathology. An 18 to 20 mm skin incision centered over the disk level of root compression is drawn to facilitate the surgical approach for a single-level procedure. For two-level procedures the incision should be planned midway between the affected levels. A stab skin incision is made with a #15 blade. A Steinmann pin or K-wire is then carefully passed through the paraspinous musculature and docked onto the lumbar lamina rostral to the level of interest. Fluoroscopic guidance is used to ensure the proper level and contact with the bony lamina to prevent introduction of the pin into the interlaminar space, where dural puncture or nerve root injury may ensue.

A series of tubular dilators with increasing diameter are inserted using lateral fluoroscopic confirmation of placement after each. Incising the fascia in addition to the skin, especially in young, muscular patients, may minimize axial force applied to each tube. Once adequate dilation is achieved, a working channel is passed and docked on the lateral aspect of the lamina where it meets the medial facet joint. The working channel is affixed to a flexible retractor arm mounted to the side of the operating table, and the tubular dilators are removed. The operative microscope is subsequently brought into the field, or an endoscope is attached to the retractor.

The lamina of interest is exposed using monopolar electrocautery to dissect away overlying soft tissue, then removed using pituitary rongeours to expose the inferolateral aspect of the rostral lamina and medial aspect of the facet joint. Once the bony anatomy is identified, a small up-angled curette is used to delineate the caudal extent of the rostral lamina and detach the affixed ligamentum flavum from its undersurface. The remainder of the operation takes place in the typical manner. A laminotomy and medial facetectomy are performed, followed by careful removal of the underlying ligamentum flavum to reveal the thecal sac and nerve root. Once the nerve root is identified, it is gently retracted medially and a diskectomy is performed in the traditional fashion. Once the disk space and neural foramen have been explored for residual fragments and adequate decompression of the nerve root is confirmed, the surgical wound is copiously irrigated with antibiotic solution. Hemostasis is achieved with a combination of bipolar electrocautery, bone wax, and application of operative hemostatic agent such as thrombin/powdered Gelfoam (Pfizer, New York, NY). The working channel is carefully removed, with inspection of muscle for bleeding, which is stopped with bipolar cautery. The wound is then closed in layers; closure of the fascia overlying the paraspinal musculature is not necessary.[6]

◆ Discussion

Traditional open lumbar laminectomy and foraminotomy for the treatment of lumbar disk herniation was first described by Mixter and Barr in 1934, then revised by Love in 1939, who proposed a method that subsequently became the gold standard for open surgical treatment of lumbar disk herniation.[7,8] This approach for single-level lumbar diskectomy involves making a 5 to 10 cm skin incision and subperiosteal dissection of the paraspinous musculature, which results in significant postoperative lumbar back pain and muscle spasm. Further, subsequent laminotomy and medial facetectomy has the potential for creating bony instability if excess pars or facet removal occurs. Chronic postoperative pain or gross instability often necessitate a subsequent lumbar fusion procedure.[1,2,9–11]

The introduction of a microsurgical technique by Yasargil and Caspar in 1977 utilizing the operating microscope offered better visualization of the operative field and reduced skin incision size and lamina resection, thereby minimizing trauma to adjacent motion segments and decreasing postoperative pain. However, the techniques of microlaminotomy and conventional laminectomy both involve subperiosteal dissection of paraspinous musculature and utilize similar style retractors, with the potential for significant postoperative back pain and muscle spasm.[12,13] The literature demonstrates that the microsurgical technique offers shorter operative time, less intraoperative blood loss, and decreased length of hospital stay with comparable patient satisfaction and long-term clinical results compared with open lumbar diskectomy.[13-16] This suggests that further reduction of incision size and muscle dissection should follow the same trends.

The minimally invasive approach for microdiskectomy utilizes a muscle-splitting tubular retractor system through which modified traditional tools and techniques of microdiskectomy for nerve root decompression may be applied. This method, first introduced by Foley and Smith in 1997, minimizes the morbidity associated with the traditional open and microscopic approaches while providing similar, if not superior, operative field visualization.[17,18] Studies comparing microscopic lumbar laminectomy have demonstrated the minimally invasive technique can result in a shorter hospital stay, less intraoperative blood loss, decreased postoperative narcotic use, and a faster return to work without a significant difference in complication rate and with similar short- and long-term clinical outcomes.[16-20] Furthermore, no significant difference in complication rate has been demonstrated compared with an open microdiskectomy.[18,21] Importantly, although minimally invasive lumbar microdiskectomy is a relatively new technique, the current literature also suggests similar short- and long-term resolution of neurological symptoms compared with the microsurgical approach for the treatment of lumbar disk herniation.[18,20-22]

The minimally invasive approach offers several key advantages over the open microsurgical approach. The diskectomy is performed through a smaller incision and without the subperiosteal dissection and lateral retraction of paraspinal musculature necessary in open microdiskectomy. This is particularly relevant in cases of multilevel disk disease, in which a longer open incision would be necessary for a microsurgical approach: in contrast, for the tubular approach, a single incision of 2 cm or less placed midway between the levels of interest may be used, followed by wanding of the tube above and below. Compared with an open approach, this technique decreases the mechanical disruption of paraspinous musculature, which has been shown to contribute to postoperative pain and muscle spasm.[18,20-22] In addition, the tubular muscle-splitting approach requires less tissue dissection overall and therefore may reduce tissue damage and residual inflammation and scarring, both of which have been shown to contribute to postoperative back pain following open lumbar laminectomy.[23-25]

In our experience, we have found particular patient populations for whom the technique of minimally invasive microdiskectomy has proven ideal. The minimization of incision size and extent of muscle dissection has implications for postoperative recovery and is of particular importance for obese and elderly patients, who commonly suffer medical comorbidities that compromise tissue integrity, impede wound healing, and decrease postoperative mobility. Established benefits of the minimally invasive approach, including decreased narcotic use in the perioperative period, decreased tissue trauma, and decreased infection rate, are especially advantageous to these patient populations. Obesity, defined as body mass index (BMI) of 30 kg/m² or greater, is a known risk factor for infectious complications in spinal surgery.[26] These patients have excess subcutaneous tissue often necessitating lengthening of a surgical incision to achieve adequate operative exposure and increasing their already heightened risk for poor postoperative wound healing and decreased mobility.[27,28] A minimally invasive tubular approach with muscle splitting facilitates soft tissue dissection and retraction, greatly decreasing the length of incision needed for adequate exposure to the relevant anatomy in obese patients (**Fig. 5.1 A–C**). A smaller incision and minimizing tissue trauma reduce subsequent scar formation and facilitate wound

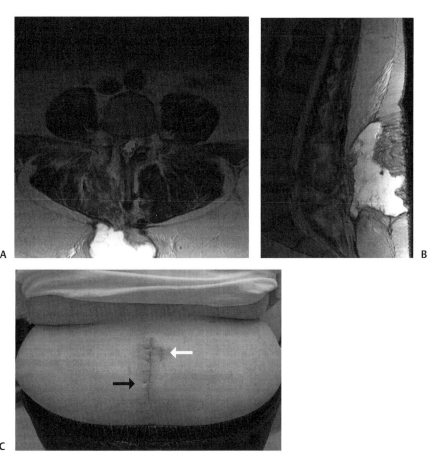

Fig. 5.1 A 47-year-old woman with a body mass index of 33 kg/m² presented with right lower extremity radiculopathy and weakness following an open L4–5 diskectomy. (**A**) Axial and (**B**) sagittal T2-weighted magnetic resonance images revealing a recurrent right L4–5 disk herniation with thecal sac and right L5 nerve root impingement, as well as extensive postoperative inflammation of the paraspinal musculature and subcutaneous fat necrosis with seroma formation. She subsequently underwent a minimally invasive right L4–5 microdiskectomy via a paramedian tubular approach. (**C**) The poorly healing large midline surgical wound from open diskectomy (black arrow) compared with the small right paramedian wound from the minimally invasive approach (white arrow).

healing, increasing postoperative mobility, which in turn decreases the risk of wound breakdown and infection in this high-risk population. A muscle-splitting approach has additional advantage in the elderly, who may have significant preoperative atrophy of the paraspinous musculature. Extensive muscular dissection can compromise blood supply and viability of the paraspinous muscle tissue, putting this patient population at risk for further tissue loss causing postoperative pain and weakness. The tubular muscle-splitting technique limits the potential for damage to paraspinal musculature and decreases blood loss, thereby optimizing postoperative recovery.[25,26,29,30]

Patients with far lateral disk herniation, in whom extensive subperiosteal muscular and bone removal would be necessary to adequately expose the disk space from a midline approach, can also benefit from the use of a muscle-sparing technique rather than an open approach. Far lateral lumbar disk herniations comprise only 2 to 12% of all lumbar herniation syndromes but are an important cause of lumbar radiculopathy. Surgical treatment can present technical challenges to the spine surgeon because of the difficulty gaining access to the far lateral compartment and the importance of the adjacent pars interarticularis and inferior facet. A midline approach to far lateral lumbar disk herniation requires wide lateral subperiosteal exposure and partial removal of one or both of these osseous structures. A paramedian approach to the lateral aspect of the disk space is thus advantageous because it directly targets the pathology while avoiding pars or facet removal. The traditional approaches still require extensive muscle dissection and retraction.[24,31,32] The use of minimal access muscle-splitting tubular dilators solves these inherent problems and is uniquely suited to these extracanalicular herniations (**Fig. 5.2**). Tubular retractor systems spare the musculature and facet joint while providing superior visualization of the neural foramen, nerve root, and intervertebral disk, thereby minimizing postoperative muscle spasm, facet instability, and trauma to neural structures.[32] The tubular approach also minimizes the extent of postoperative scar formation, thereby providing greater likelihood of clinical symptom improvement given that some

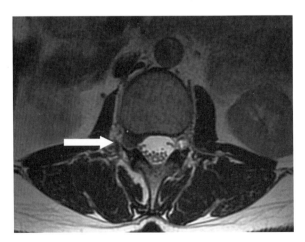

Fig. 5.2 Axial T2-weighted magnetic resonance imaging revealing a far lateral disk herniation (*white arrow*) ideally suited for a minimally invasive approach.

authors propose fibrosis and scar formation may play a role in continued or recurrent radicular pain after diskectomy.[24] For cases of far lateral disk herniation, an incision is made ~4 cm lateral to the midline. A Steinmann pin is docked on the junction of the transverse process and pars of the cephalad vertebral level under fluoroscopic guidance. The musculature is split with dilators, and the working channel is then directed caudad toward the diseased disk space. Voyadzis et al recently reviewed 20 of their patients with far lateral disk herniations who were treated by a minimally invasive approach.[33] Fourteen of 20 had an excellent outcome, and the remaining six had a good outcome according to the MacNab criteria, with an average length of hospital stay of 8 hours and an estimated blood loss of 30 mL.[33]

The minimally invasive approach may also be advantageous in patients who have previously undergone lumbar diskectomy or laminectomy and suffer a recurrent disk herniation. Reports of recurrent lumbar disk herniation after prior lumbar diskectomy range from 1 to 27% depending on the method of measurement and length of follow-up.[34–37] For these patients reoperation is often necessary due to persistent debilitating radicular pain or neurological deficit. However, the formation of scar tissue after a prior operation can mask traditional anatomical landmarks, making future surgical dissection more challenging and increasing the likelihood of durotomy, nerve root injury, and failure to relieve symptoms, with an increase in postoperative pain and a need for additional operation.[36,38,39] Dissection through muscular scar tissue formed after a previous diskectomy may be avoided in these patients by using a separate, more lateral incision and directly targeting the pathology with a minimally invasive approach. By utilizing a tubular retraction system, a working channel is docked directly on the facet of the disk space of interest through naive tissue, effectively converting a potentially difficult reoperative case into a more straightforward one (**Fig. 5.3**). Developing a plane between scarred muscle from a prior operation and the medial aspect of the facet is very straightforward using a straight curette through a tubular retractor. Multiple studies have reported comparable clinical results with minimally invasive lumbar diskectomy for recurrent disk herniation when compared with microdiskectomy, with no additional risk of complication.[36,37,39–41] Any surgeon who has gone through previously operated paraspinous muscle exposed via subperiosteal exposure knows firsthand that fibrosis and scarring of the muscle is extensive and can hamper subsequent operations. Several studies evaluating the paraspinal musculature after minimally invasive diskectomy have demonstrated decreased scarring, fibrosis, and atrophy.[23–25]

There are patient populations in whom we would favor an open diskectomy to a minimally invasive microsurgical approach. In a young, thin, healthy individual with single-level disk disease, open microdiskectomy may be equivalent to a tubular approach. Specifically, we have found that patients with a skin to facet distance of less than 4 cm in the sagittal plane on MRI can experience extensive muscle creep with the use of currently available tubular retractors. In these cases, a traditional microdiskectomy may be more suitable. Surgeons with extensive experience using tubular retractors can perform limited subperiosteal dissection with the tubular retractor to help decrease muscle creep. Arts et al recently performed a double-blinded, randomized, controlled trial comparing single-level minimally invasive lumbar microdiskectomy to traditional open microdiskectomy for patients with lumbar radiculopathy. In this well-designed and methodologically sound study the authors found that there

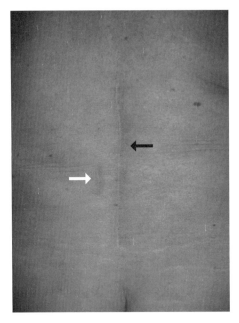

Fig. 5.3 A 56-year-old man who previously underwent an open multilevel lumbar laminectomy for stenosis (black arrow) developed an acute left L4–5 disk herniation treated with a minimally invasive tubular retractor using a paramedian incision to avoid scar tissue (white arrow).

was no significant difference in postoperative outcome or recovery time between the two treatment groups.[42] The amount of experience of the surgeons performing the minimally invasive arm of the study was not clearly defined. Patients with recurrent disk herniation or significant comorbidities were excluded from this study, and the average BMI in patients undergoing tubular versus conventional microdiskectomy was 26.0 and 25.4, respectively. Of note, Arts et al used a midline approach for both the tubular and the open arms, thus requiring subperiosteal muscle dissection in both techniques. Previous randomized, controlled trials comparing muscle-splitting tubular diskectomy via a paramedian incision with conventional microdiskectomy have found decreased postoperative analgesia and shorter hospital stay in the minimally invasive groups.[18,21,43]

◆ Conclusion

Minimally invasive microdiskectomy is an effective surgical approach for treatment of lower-extremity radiculopathy secondary to single or dual level lumbar disk herniation. This approach provides access to disk pathology using a smaller skin incision and muscle-splitting technique with minimal bony dissection, resulting in reduced postoperative back pain and muscle spasm, preservation of adjacent motion segments, and decreased length of hospital stay. These characteristics make this approach ideal for treatment of far lateral disk herniation and recurrent disk herniation in obese and elderly patients. In cases of thin, young, healthy patients, the open and minimally invasive approach for lumbar microdiskectomy may be equivalent.

References

1. Weber H. The natural history of disc herniation and the influence of intervention. Spine (Phila Pa 1976) 1994;19:2234–2238

2. Yorimitsu E, Chiba K, Toyama Y, Hirabayashi K. Long-term outcomes of standard discectomy for lumbar disc herniation: a follow-up study of more than 10 years. Spine (Phila Pa 1976) 2001;26:652–657

3. Perez-Cruet MJ, Fessler RG, Perin NI. Review: complications of minimally invasive spinal surgery. Neurosurgery 2002;51(5, Suppl):S26–S36

4. Le H, Sandhu FA, Fessler RG. Clinical outcomes after minimal-access surgery for recurrent lumbar disc herniation. Neurosurg Focus 2003;15:E12

5. Fessler RG, Khoo LT. Minimally invasive cervical microendoscopic foraminotomy: an initial clinical experience. Neurosurgery 2002;51(5, Suppl):S37–S45

6. Foley KT, Smith MM, Rampersaud YR. Microendoscopic discectomy. In: Operative Neurosurgical Techniques, eds. Schmidek and Sweet. Philadelphia, PA: WB Saunders; 1995:2246–2256

7. Love JG. Removal of protruded intervertebral disc without laminectomy. Proc Staff Meet Mayo Clin 1939;14:800–805

8. Mixter WJ, Barr JS. Rupture of the intervertebral disc with involvement of the spinal canal. N Engl J Med 1934;211:210–215

9. Abramovitz JN, Neff SR. Lumbar disc surgery: results of the Prospective Lumbar Discectomy Study of the Joint Section on Disorders of the Spine and Peripheral Nerves of the American Association of Neurological Surgeons and the Congress of Neurological Surgeons. Neurosurgery 1991;29:301–307

10. Daneyemez M, Sali A, Kahraman S, Beduk A, Seber N. Outcome analyses in 1072 surgically treated lumbar disc herniations. Minim Invasive Neurosurg 1999;42:63–68

11. Davis RA. A long-term outcome analysis of 984 surgically treated herniated lumbar discs. J Neurosurg 1994;80:415–421

12. Caspar W. A new surgical procedure for lumbar disc herniation causing less tissue damage through a microsurgical approach. In: Advances in Neurosurgery, eds. Wollenweber, Brock, Hamer, Klinger, Spoerri. Berlin, Germany: Springer-Verlag; 1997:74–77

13. Caspar W, Campbell B, Barbier DD, Kretschmmer R, Gotfried Y. The Caspar microsurgical discectomy and comparison with a conventional standard lumbar disc procedure. Neurosurgery 1991;28:78–86

14. Findlay GF, Hall BI, Musa BS, Oliveira MD, Fear SC. A 10-year follow-up of the outcome of lumbar microdiscectomy. Spine (Phila Pa 1976) 1998;23:1168–1171

15. Türeyen K. One-level one-sided lumbar disc surgery with and without microscopic assistance: 1-year outcome in 114 consecutive patients. J Neurosurg 2003;99(3, Suppl):247–250

16. Katayama Y, Matsuyama Y, Yoshihara H, et al. Comparison of surgical outcomes between macro discectomy and micro discectomy for lumbar disc herniation: a prospective randomized study with surgery performed by the same spine surgeon. J Spinal Disord Tech 2006;19:344–347

17. Perez-Cruet MJ, Foley KT, Isaacs RE, et al. Microendoscopic lumbar discectomy: technical note. Neurosurgery 2002;51(5, Suppl):S129–S136

18. Righesso O, Falavigna A, Avanzi O. Comparison of open discectomy with microendoscopic discectomy in lumbar disc herniations: results of a randomized controlled trial. Neurosurgery 2007;61:545–549

19. Muramatsu K, Hachiya Y, Morita C. Postoperative magnetic resonance imaging of lumbar disc herniation: comparison of microendoscopic discectomy and Love's method. Spine (Phila Pa 1976) 2001;26:1599–1605

20. Palmer S. Use of a tubular retractor system in microscopic lumbar discectomy: 1 year prospective results in 135 patients. Neurosurg Focus 2002;13:E5

21. Ryang YM, Oertel MF, Mayfrank L, Gilsbach JM, Rohde V. Standard open microdiscectomy versus minimal access trocar microdiscectomy: results of a prospective randomized study. Neurosurgery 2008;62:174–181

22. German JW, Adamo MA, Hoppenot RG, Blossom JH, Nagle HA. Perioperative results following lumbar discectomy: comparison of minimally invasive discectomy and standard microdiscectomy. Neurosurg Focus 2008;25:E20

23. Huang TJ, Hsu RW, Li YY, Cheng CC. Less systemic cytokine response in patients following microendoscopic versus open lumbar discectomy. J Orthop Res 2005;23:406–411

24. Almeida DB, Prandini MN, Awamura Y, et al. Outcome following lumbar disc surgery: the role of fibrosis. Acta Neurochir (Wien) 2008;150:1167–1176

25. Lee SH, Chung SE, Ahn Y, Kim TH, Park JY, Shin SW. Comparative radiologic evaluation of percutaneous endoscopic lumbar discectomy and open microdiscectomy: a matched cohort analysis. Mt Sinai J Med 2006;73:795–801

26. Patel N, Bagan B, Vadera S, et al. Obesity and spine surgery: relation to perioperative complications. J Neurosurg Spine 2007;6:291–297

27. Cole JS IV, Jackson TR. Minimally invasive lumbar discectomy in obese patients. Neurosurgery 2007;61:539–544

28. Rosen DS, Ferguson SD, Ogden AT, Huo D, Fessler RG. Obesity and self-reported outcome after minimally invasive lumbar spinal fusion surgery. Neurosurgery 2008;63:956–960

29. Rosen DS, O'Toole JE, Eichholz KM, et al. Minimally invasive lumbar spinal decompression in the elderly: outcomes of 50 patients aged 75 years and older. Neurosurgery 2007;60:503–509

30. Shin DA, Kim KN, Shin HC, Yoon H. The efficacy of microendoscopic discectomy in reducing iatrogenic muscle injury. J Neurosurg Spine 2008;8:39–43

31. Tessitore E, de Tribolet N. Far-lateral lumbar disc herniation: the microsurgical transmuscular approach. Neurosurgery 2004;54:939–942

32. Kotil K, Akcetin M, Bilge T. A minimally invasive transmuscular approach to far-lateral L5–S1 level disc herniations: a prospective study. J Spinal Disord Tech 2007;20:132–138

33. Voyadzis JM, Gala VC, Sandhu FA, Fessler RG. Minimally invasive approach for far lateral disc herniations: results from 20 patients. Minimally Invasive Neurosurgery 2010. In press.

34. Watters WC III, McGirt MJ. An evidence-based review of the literature on the consequences of conservative versus aggressive discectomy for the treatment of primary disc herniation with radiculopathy. Spine J 2009;9:240–257

35. McGirt MJ, Ambrossi GL, Datoo G, et al. Recurrent disc herniation and long-term back pain after primary lumbar discectomy: review of outcomes reported for limited versus aggressive disc removal. Neurosurgery 2009;64:338–344

36. Isaacs RE, Podichetty V, Fessler RG. Microendoscopic discectomy for recurrent disc herniations. Neurosurg Focus 2003;15:E11

37. Le H, Sandhu FA, Fessler RG. Clinical outcomes after minimal-access surgery for recurrent lumbar disc herniation. Neurosurg Focus 2003;15:E12

38. Suk KS, Lee HM, Moon SH, Kim NH. Recurrent lumbar disc herniation: results of operative management. Spine (Phila Pa 1976) 2001;26:672–676

39. Ahn Y, Lee SH, Park WM, Lee HY, Shin SW, Kang HY. Percutaneous endoscopic lumbar discectomy for recurrent disc herniation: surgical technique, outcome, and prognostic factors of 43 consecutive cases. Spine (Phila Pa 1976) 2004;29:E326–E332

40. Hoogland T, van den Brekel-Dijkstra K, Schubert M, Miklitz B. Endoscopic transforaminal discectomy for recurrent lumbar disc herniation: a prospective, cohort evaluation of 262 consecutive cases. Spine (Phila Pa 1976) 2008;33:973–978

41. Swartz KR, Trost GR. Recurrent lumbar disc herniation. Neurosurg Focus 2003;15:E10

42. Arts MP, Brand R, van den Akker ME, Koes BW, Bartels RH, Peul WC; Leiden-The Hague Spine Intervention Prognostic Study Group (SIPS). Tubular diskectomy vs conventional microdiskectomy for sciatica: a randomized controlled trial. JAMA 2009;302:149–158

43. Brock M, Kunkel P, Papavero L. Lumbar microdiscectomy: subperiosteal versus transmuscular approach and influence on the early postoperative analgesic consumption. Eur Spine J 2008;17:518–522

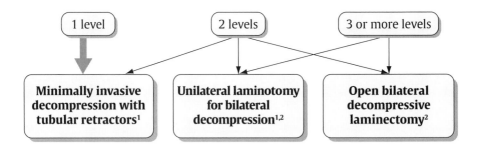

[1]The preservation of posterior osteoligamentous structures afforded by these may diminish the potential for iatrogenic instability particularly in patients with underlying spondylolisthesis or scoliosis who are not candidates for fusion.

[2]The traditional midline subperiosteal exposure may be more appropriate for thin patients owing to the difficulty in dilating through the paraspinal musculature and subsequent muscle creep hampering visualization through the tubular retractor.

6

Minimally Invasive Lumbar Laminectomy for Stenosis

Sathish J. Subbaiah, Richard G. Fessler, Jean-Marc Voyadzis, and Faheem A. Sandhu

Lumbar spinal stenosis is defined as any condition that leads to narrowing of the spinal canal and exiting nerve roots. It can be divided into six categories, as defined by Arnoldi et al and modified by Katz and Harris.[1,2] These include congenital stenosis, acquired stenosis, iatrogenic stenosis, spondylotic stenosis, and posttraumatic stenosis. Most frequently, stenosis is caused by a constellation of factors that are associated with lumbar degenerative disease. Anterior to the neural canal, the degenerating lumbar disks continue to desiccate and lose their elasticity. This then leads to loss of lumbar disk height and a broad "bulging" of the disk contents into the neural canal, and laterally into the lateral recess and neural foramen. Lateral to the central neural canal, chronic stress and strain on the lumbar facets lead to hypertrophy of these joints and often the formation of osteophytes and degenerative cysts. These enlarged, overgrown facets also contribute to pressure on the exiting nerve roots and diminish the entire cross-sectional area of the lumbar canal. Degenerative changes also lead to the hypertrophy of the ligamentum flavum in the dorsal aspect of the spinal canal. Furthermore, as the overall disk height collapses anteriorly, the ligamentum flavum begins to buckle and impinge upon the neural canal as well. When the patient extends the spine, the posterior elements are compressed, exacerbating the buckling of the ligamentum flavum and leading to worsening of the clinical symptoms.

Patients with congenital stenosis will often present before the age of 65, usually in their 30s to 40s. These patients are born with congenitally shortened pedicles leading to a narrowed cross-sectional area of the lumbar canal from birth. Degenerative changes in the lumbar disk and facets are not tolerated well and lead to early presentation of neurological symptoms. Iatrogenic stenosis can be the result of laminectomy or lumbar fusion. There is evidence that in a small percentage of the population, fusion of the lumbar motion segments will lead to accelerated degenerative changes at the levels above and below the fusion.[3]

◆ Preoperative Evaluation

The ideal candidate for surgery of lumbar stenosis is the elderly patient with classic symptoms of lumbar claudication who has failed a thorough trial of nonsurgical therapy. These patients complain of back and bilateral buttock pain that has severely limited their ability to walk. This pain can often radiate into the thighs and legs in various dermatomal distributions. Pain in the bilateral buttock region that is exacerbated with standing or walking and gradually relieved by sitting is classical neurogenic claudication. The pain can be initiated by the transition from a sitting to a standing position, but often it begins after a short period of standing or ambulating. The pain is often described as worsened with extension of the spine and mildly relieved by flexion of the spine. This "shopping cart" sign, where patients will describe symptomatic relief while walking in a flexed position with the aid of a walker or shopping cart, is helpful in identifying patients with lumbar stenosis. A detailed history can help differentiate neurogenic claudication from vascular claudication. In vascular claudication, patients do not generally describe significant pain with standing. They often describe pain that is initiated with walking, especially uphill, that is immediately relieved by rest. Patients with vascular claudication will also reproduce their pain with exercise on a bicycle, whereas patients with lumbar stenosis will often not be able to reproduce their back pain in the flexed bicycle riding position.

To confirm the diagnosis, all patients with these complaints should have anteroposterior (AP), lateral, flexion, and extension x-rays of their lumbar spine. These films quickly identify the extent of degenerative changes in the lumbar spine, the overall sagittal and coronal balance, the degree of disk height loss, end plate sclerosis, and facet hypertrophy. Furthermore, these radiographs can rule out the presence of spondylolisthesis and the presence of any abnormal motion between the lumbar levels. The presence or absence of motion can be a key component in the treatment algorithm for lumbar stenosis. The next radiographic test that is ordered is magnetic resonance imaging (MRI) or computed tomographic (CT) myelography in patients who are unable to undergo MRI. Although the CT-myelogram gives a better understanding of the bony anatomy and a clearer view of facet hypertrophy, it is an invasive procedure with an associated risk of complications. MRI will give a clear view of the soft tissue anatomy, including the degree of degenerative changes in the lumbar disks and ligamentum flavum. There is often a complete loss of T2 cerebrospinal fluid (CSF) signal at the level of the most severe lumbar stenosis (**Fig. 6.1A,B**). The classic appearance of a "trefoil"-shaped lumbar canal can also be appreciated on axial T2 MRI sequences. This trefoil shape is the result of compromise of the cross-sectional area by the degenerated, bulging lumbar disks anteriorly, the hypertrophic facets laterally, and the buckling enlarged ligamentum flavum posteriorly. The MRI can also reveal the presence of degenerative facet cysts, "synovial cysts," that can further lead to canal narrowing. MRI scans can be highly sensitive in identifying the cardinal radiographic signs of lumbar stenosis. It is important to clearly correlate the findings on the history and physical with the radiographic results. In one study performed on asymptomatic patients, the presence of lumbar stenosis identified on MRI was as high as 20%.[4]

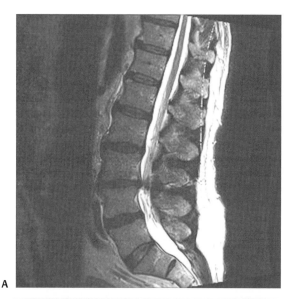

A

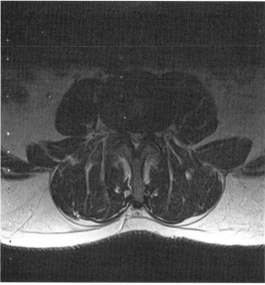

B

Fig. 6.1 **(A)** Sagittal and **(B)** axial T2-weighted magnetic resonance imaging showing lumbar stenosis at L3–4 ideally suited for a minimally invasive approach.

◆ Open Decompressive Laminectomy

Recent prospective, randomized, multicentered studies have demonstrated a significantly better outcome for the surgical treatment of lumbar stenosis over nonsurgical treatment.[5] The classic surgical treatment of lumbar stenosis is an open posterior decompressive lumbar laminectomy. This is performed via a midline incision over the affected lumbar levels. The midline lumbodorsal fascia is incised the length of the skin incision, and periosteal dissection is used to strip the erector spinae musculature off the posterior spinal elements. These denervated muscles are retracted laterally throughout the procedure. The supraspinous ligament and interspinal ligaments are then resected with the spinous processes. The bilateral lamina, medial facet joint complexes, and ligamentum flavum are then removed. Upon adequate visualization of the decompressed lumbar canal and exiting nerve roots, hemostasis is achieved and the wound is closed. The stripped paraspinal musculature is reapproximated with loose sutures. The thoracodorsal fascia is closed watertight, followed by closure of the subdermal layer. There are many studies that have shown the effectiveness of this operation to treat lumbar stenosis.[6,7] However, the disadvantages of this procedure were also clearly evident to many observers.

The first major disadvantage of the open technique is the muscle injury that results from the dissection, denervation, and retraction. The second major disadvantage is the destabilization that results from the disruption of the supraspinal and interspinal ligaments. The third disadvantage is the potential destabilization that occurs with significant bilateral medial facetectomies that are often performed. Finally, the frequency of medical complications in the elderly population during the recovery time required for the open procedure can also pose a problem.

◆ Unilateral Laminotomy for Bilateral Decompression

There have been several steps in the evolution of less invasive treatment of lumbar stenosis. An open procedure with bilateral laminoforaminotomies was first advocated to preserve the posterior tension band.[8] This was followed by the recommendation for a less invasive unilateral open laminoforaminotomy to achieve a bilateral decompression while preserving the contralateral musculature.[9] This approach involves a midline incision, unilateral subperiosteal exposure, ipsilateral laminotomy and medial facetectomy, and contralateral decompression by undercutting the lamina from within the spinal canal with the use of the operating microscope. The operating table can be tilted away from the surgeon to provide greater visualization for performing the contralateral decompression. This technique preserves the posterior tension band, contralateral facet joints, and contralateral musculature. In a retrospective review of 374 patients with spinal stenosis treated with unilateral laminotomy and bilateral microdecompression, Costa et al found 87.9% of patients experienced a significant benefit with a very low complication rate.[10] No patient went on to require a fusion procedure for iatrogenic instability.

◆ Minimally Invasive Decompression

Two major technological advancements pioneered modern minimally invasive spinal surgery. First, the introduction of the tubular retraction system allowed for an effective muscle-sparing access to the spine. Second, the advancement in microscopic and endoscopic technology allowed for a safe, illuminated, and magnified view of the pathological conditions that could now be treated.

In 2002, a novel minimally invasive laminectomy was presented and quickly validated in clinical series. The microendoscopic decompression of stenosis (MEDS) offers an alternative to the classic open laminectomy. The MEDS accomplishes the same goals as the open laminectomy procedure, the decompression of the lumbar canal and exiting nerve roots, without the major drawbacks of an open procedure. The surgical techniques are described in detail.

The patient is given preoperative antibiotics and brought into the operating room and induced with general endotracheal anesthesia. Paralytics are not routinely administered because it is beneficial to observe any spontaneous activity while decompressing the exiting nerve roots. A Foley catheter is not routinely placed for this procedure. The patient is positioned prone on a radiolucent Wilson frame on a Jackson table. The Wilson frame is then fully elevated allowing for further distraction of the laminae and facets during the decompression. All the pressure points are well padded, the neck is maintained throughout the positioning and procedure in a neutral position, and the eyes are visibly free of any pressure. The patient is prepped and draped, and the clamp for the tubular retraction system (such as the METRx system, Medtronic, Minneapolis, MN) is affixed to the bed at the level of the hip. The fluoroscopic C-arm is sterilely draped and brought into position to obtain an AP view of the lumbar spine. The operative level is marked and a vertical line is drawn 1.5 cm lateral to midline on the operative side. The base of the C-arm is placed opposite to the surgeon. The C-arm is then positioned to obtain lateral images of the spine.

The operative level is once again checked in the lateral position, and the local anesthetic with epinephrine is injected. A small stab incision is made, and the Steinmann pin is passed down to the medial bony facet. By passing the Steinmann pin lateral to midline directly onto the medial facet, the risk of passing the wire into the interlaminar space is minimized. The fluoroscopic image confirms the proper working trajectory. After this confirmation, the incision is extended 1 cm above and below the Steinmann pin. A set of serial dilators are passed over the Steinmann pin. The dilators are introduced with a firm downward pressure combined with a rotating motion. The goal is to split the paraspinal muscle fibers. After passage of the first dilator, the Steinmann pin is removed. As larger dilators are introduced, the slight medial angulation of the dilators is performed to assume the final working position. Fluoroscopy is used to confirm that the dilators are resting on the bony facet and lamina. An 18 or 20 mm final working channel is passed over the final dilator and secured to the flexible arm clamped to the table (**Fig. 6.2**). The endoscope is white balanced, focused, and attached to the tubular retractor in a friction coupling device. Alternatively, an operating microscope can be used to perform the procedure and has the advantage of superior optics with three-dimensional views. The disadvantage of the microscope lies in the awkward angles that it must assume to follow the various movements of the working channel that can lead to surgeon discomfort.

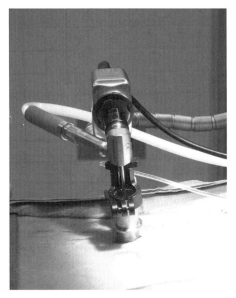

Fig. 6.2 Tubular dilator with attached endoscope fixed in operative position.

The next stage of the procedure is to clear the remaining soft tissue off the medial facet and lamina with the Bovie electrocautery. After the margins of the lamina are defined, a small straight and angled curette is used to dissect the ligamentum flavum away from the lamina and medial facet. It is important to carefully dissect the ligament and dura away from the bone prior to beginning the laminotomy. The laminotomy is begun at the inferior laminar edge and continued rostrally to the level of the pedicle with an angled Kerrison rongeur. The lateral edge of the lamina and medial facet complex are removed with the Kerrison rongeur as well after dissecting away the underlying ligamentum flavum. In patients with severely hypertrophied facets, a drill is used (e.g., AM8, Midas Rex Institute, Fort Worth, TX) to thin the facet and lamina prior to removal with the Kerrison. The lateral bony decompression is extended down to the neuroforamen to achieve an adequate decompression of the ipsilateral traverse nerve root. The ligamentum flavum is not removed at this point of the procedure because it protects the underlying dura and nerve root.

After adequate decompression of the lamina, medial facet, and neural foramen, the working channel is angled medially to expose the undersurface of the spinous process and contralateral lamina. This wanding motion, combined with the 30 degree viewing angle of the endoscope, allows for good visualization of the contralateral decompression. If a microscope is used, the operating table can be tilted contralaterally to improve the viewing angle. The drill is once again used to carefully drill the undersurface of the spinous process. The ligamentum flavum is thin at this medial point and a specialized drill with a protective guard can be used to protect the dura. The drilling is continued to the undersurface of the contralateral lamina, once again retaining the ligamentum flavum to protect the dura. Through the combined use of the drill and Kerrison rongeurs, the decompression can be extended to the contralateral lateral recess and neural foramen. Bone wax is used liberally on all resected bone surfaces to help with hemostasis.

After completing the bony decompression, attention is turned to carefully remove the ligamentum flavum. The endoscope is repositioned back to its original operative position. A blunt nerve hook or angled curette is used to carefully dissect the ligament off the dura. The ligament is thinnest at its rostral and medial point. The ligamentum flavum overlying the dura, in the lateral recess, and overlying the neural foramen is carefully removed with the Kerrison rongeurs. The endoscope is then positioned to view the contralateral ligamentum flavum and the procedure is repeated. Prior to removing this ligament, it is very important to carefully dissect it free from the underlying dura to avoid a CSF leak or neural injury. A small blunt nerve hook is used to assess the decompression in the bilateral neural foramen. The dura is then visually inspected to be free from any compression from the rostral to caudal pedicle (**Fig. 6.3**). After hemostasis is achieved, the wound is irrigated with antibiotic saline. The tubular retractor system is carefully removed, taking care to visually inspect the muscle and fascial layers during removal to identify any bleeding sources, which are cauterized with bipolar cautery. The fascia and skin are closed in the standard fashion, and the skin is closed with Dermabond (Ethicon, Inc., Somerville, NJ).

In cases with two levels of pathology, a single incision can be made at the midpoint of the two working levels, and the working channel is wanded cephalad or caudad. A separate tissue path may also be dilated through the same incision to complete the decompression at each level.

The MEDS technique was originally developed in a cadaveric model and was confirmed via CT to have a level of decompression of the lumbar canal similar to open

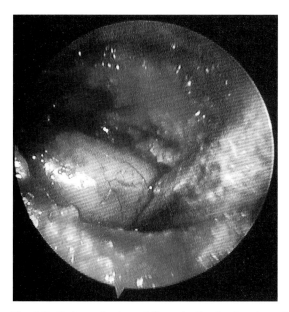

Fig. 6.3 Endoscopic view of the pulsating lumbar dura at the completion of the microendoscopic decompression of stenosis (MEDS) procedure. The Kerrison rongeur is used to remove the overlying ligamentum flavum.

procedures.[11] Multiple clinical series have compared the results of the MEDS procedure to open laminotomy. In the first such study, 25 patients were treated with open decompressive laminectomy, and their results were compared with 25 patients who underwent the MEDS procedure. The results revealed similar effectiveness of the procedures. In the MEDS group, 16% reported resolution of their back pain, 68% reported improvement of their back pain symptoms, and 16% reported no change in their symptoms.[12] This study also revealed less estimated blood loss (EBL) (68 mL vs 193 mL), postoperative stay (42 h vs 94 h), and less narcotic use in the MEDS group as compared with the open laminotomy group. In this initial study the operative time was longer (109 min./level vs 88 min./level) in the MEDS group. In a more recent review, 48 patients underwent MEDS and their results were compared with a historical cohort of 32 patients who underwent an open decompression. This review also reproduced the results of decreased operative blood loss, postoperative hospital stay, postoperative pain, and narcotic usage.[13] In this review 32 of the 48 patients were followed for 4 years postop; 88% of these patients continued to report improvements of their symptoms at 4 years. Other published clinical series have also recently reported very favorable outcomes.[14–16]

Once comfortable with the MEDS technique, the approach offers significant other advantages over the standard open lumbar laminectomy without sacrificing the operative goals of surgery—decompression of the lumbar canal and nerve roots.[12,17] The MEDS approach utilizes a unilateral muscle dilation approach to visualize the lamina and medial facet complex. There is no stripping, devascularizing, or denervating the paraspinal musculature to access the lumbar spine. This leads to significant differences in blood loss and postoperative pain between the two procedures. The diminished need for narcotics can lead to earlier mobilization of the patients as well as faster recuperation from surgery, earlier discharge from the hospital, and earlier return to normal activities.

Postoperative stability of the lumbar spine has increasingly been shown to correlate favorably with clinical outcomes. MEDS preserves stability after surgery for lumbar stenosis,[18] presumably by preserving the contralateral musculature, and the supraspinous and interspinous ligaments, vital components of the "posterior tension band," which play a significant role in stability of the lumbar spine. For the classic open decompressive laminectomy, the reoperation rate was 5% at 2 years and 11% at 10 years in one study of 9664 patients.[19] Although more clinical studies are needed to verify long-term results, preliminary data suggest a much lower reoperation rate for MEDS.

Muscle atrophy following MEDS has been shown to be significantly less than with open decompression of stenosis. Furthermore, physiological stress hormones are significantly lower in patients undergoing minimally invasive surgical procedures compared with open procedures.[20,21] This leads to fewer complications in "high-risk" patients, such as octogenarians[22] and morbidly obese patients.[23] Finally, another advantage of MEDS over conventional open decompression of stenosis is that infection rates are significantly lower.[24]

◆ Discussion

The decision to pursue a minimally invasive approach using tubular retractors as opposed to a traditional midline subperiosteal exposure for lumbar stenosis depends on the following factors: extent of disease (i.e., number of levels), presence of concomitant spondylolisthesis or scoliosis, body habitus or mass index (BMI), and surgeon experience. Patients with central stenosis at one or two levels can be treated minimally invasively using the same 2 cm incision with wanding of the working channel cephalad or caudad (**Fig. 6.1A,B**). Three-level stenosis requires a separate incision and separate dilation through the paraspinal musculature. Two separate dilations have the potential to cause a greater degree of postoperative pain and muscle spasm. It may also extend the length of the surgery significantly when compared with the traditional approach. For these reasons, elderly patients with multilevel stenosis without spondylolisthesis or significant scoliosis may be best managed with a midline subperiosteal approach (**Fig. 6.4A–C**).

Patients with severe stenosis and a concomitant low-grade, nonmobile spondylolisthesis or scoliosis who are not appropriate for fusion are ideal candidates for a minimally invasive decompression given that the integrity of the posterior osteoligamentous structures is maintained (**Fig. 6.5A-D**). This should lessen the potential for iatrogenic instability.[14] If the disease process spans more than two levels, a unilateral laminotomy and bilateral microscopic decompression may be a good option. This approach preserves the posterior tension band and contralateral facet joints and may be more efficient in the setting of multilevel disease when compared with the use of two incisions and separate dilations with tubular retractors.

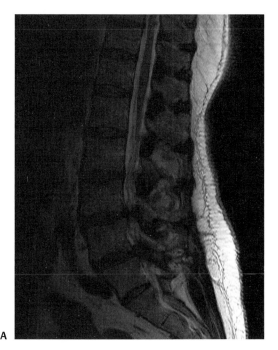

A

Fig. 6.4 A 67-year-old lady developed profound foot weakness. Sagittal **(A)** and axial T2 MRI showing critical stenosis at L3–4.

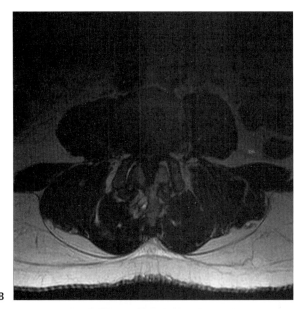

B

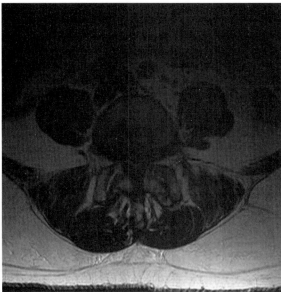

C

Fig. 6.4 (*continued*)   **(B)** And L4–5. **(C)** Dynamic x-rays showed normal alignment without instability. She underwent an open decompressive laminectomy with complete resolution of her symptoms.

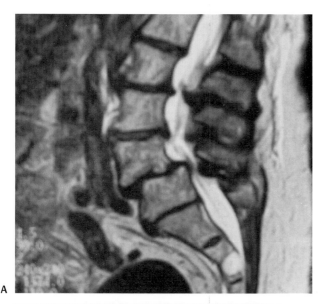

A

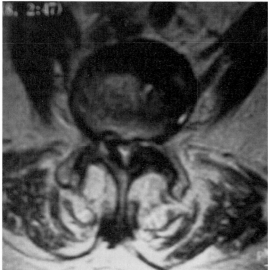

B

Fig. 6.5 An 86-year-old woman with an extensive past medical history developed severe neurogenic claudication. She had no back pain. **(A)** Sagittal and **(B)** axial T2-weighted magnetic resonance imaging demonstrated a grade 2 L4–5 spondylolisthesis with severe stenosis. Flexion and extension lumbar spine x-rays demonstrated no movement. She underwent a minimally invasive decompressive laminectomy with complete resolution of her leg pain. Follow-up dynamic x-rays revealed no iatrogenic instability at 1-year follow-up.

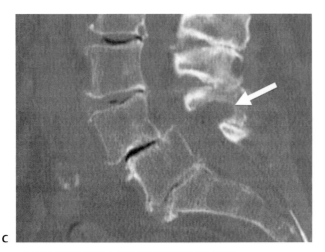

C

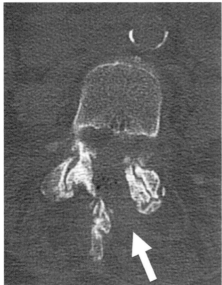

D

Fig. 6.5 (*continued*) **(C)** Postoperative sagittal and **(D)** axial computed tomography demonstrating the minimally invasive decompression (*white arrows*).

Body habitus or patient girth may also influence the decision-making process. Thin patients with a skin to facet joint distance of less than 4 cm measured in a sagittal or axial plane may not be appropriate for the use of tubular retractors, where a significant amount of muscle creep may be encountered, limiting visualization. Conversely, obese patients are ideally suited for a minimally invasive approach because of the reduction of tissue dissection and incision size that it affords.[24]

Those surgeons not comfortable with minimally invasive surgical techniques may elect open surgery. Another argument that favors open surgery is the learning curve associated with minimally invasive techniques. However, operative times for MEDS, although initially longer, shorten with experience to less time than that required for open surgery. Moreover, after learning an initial procedure, adding other minimally invasive techniques becomes progressively easier. The unilateral approach with bilateral microscopic decompression is a technique that transitions from the open laminectomy to the microendoscopic laminectomy with tubular retractors requiring a far shorter learning curve.

◆ Conclusion

Lumbar stenosis is a very common disease process that will be encountered by the practicing spine surgeon. It is the authors' belief that the MEDS approach offers improved results compared with the open decompressive laminectomy without the significant disadvantages of the open procedure for one- or two-level disease The major disadvantage of the minimally invasive surgery is the learning curve required to master the techniques. As more surgeons become familiar with minimally invasive decompression, only a few simple modifications are needed to develop proficiency in this technique. For extensive multilevel disease, a midline subperiosteal exposure and decompression may be more appropriate. The preservation of the posterior tension band and contralateral structures afforded by the unilateral approach to a bilateral decompression significantly lowers the potential for instability.

References

1. Arnoldi CC, Brodsky AE, Cauchoix J, et al. Lumbar spinal stenosis and nerve root entrapment syndromes: definition and classification. Clin Orthop Relat Res 1976;(115):4–5
2. Katz JN, Harris MB. Clinical practice: lumbar spinal stenosis. N Engl J Med 2008;358:818–825
3. Park P, Garton HJ, Gala VC, Hoff JT, McGillicuddy JE. Adjacent segment disease after lumbar or lumbosacral fusion: review of the literature. Spine (Phila Pa 1976) 2004;29:1938–1944
4. Jensen MC, Brant-Zawadzki MN, Obuchowski N, Modic MT, Malkasian D, Ross JS. Magnetic resonance imaging of the lumbar spine in people without back pain. N Engl J Med 1994;331:69–73
5. Weinstein JN, Tosteson TD, Lurie JD, et al; SPORT Investigators. Surgical versus nonsurgical therapy for lumbar spinal stenosis. N Engl J Med 2008;358:794–810
6. Jönsson B, Annertz M, Sjöberg C, Strömqvist B. A prospective and consecutive study of surgically treated lumbar spinal stenosis, II: Five-year follow-up by an independent observer. Spine (Phila Pa 1976) 1997;22:2938–2944
7. Cirak B, Alptekin M, Palaoglu S, Ozcan OE, Ozgen T. Surgical therapy for lumbar spinal stenosis: evaluation of 300 cases. Neurosurg Rev 2001;24:80–82
8. Joson RM, McCormick KJ. Preservation of the supraspinous ligament for spinal stenosis: a technical note. Neurosurgery 1987;21:420–422
9. Spetzger U, Bertalanffy H, Reinges MH, Gilsbach JM. Unilateral laminotomy for bilateral decompression of lumbar spinal stenosis, II: Clinical experiences. Acta Neurochir (Wien) 1997;139:397–403
10. Costa F, Sassi M, Cardia A, et al. Degenerative lumbar spinal stenosis: analysis of results in a series of 374 patients treated with unilateral laminotomy for bilateral microdecompression. J Neurosurg Spine 2007;7:579–586

11. Guiot BH, Khoo LT, Fessler RG. A minimally invasive technique for decompression of the lumbar spine. Spine (Phila Pa 1976) 2002;27:432–438

12. Khoo LT, Fessler RG. Microendoscopic decompressive laminotomy for the treatment of lumbar stenosis. Neurosurgery 2002;51(5, Suppl):S146–S154

13. Asgarzadie F, Khoo LT. Minimally invasive operative management for lumbar spinal stenosis: overview of early and long-term outcomes. Orthop Clin North Am 2007;38:387–399, abstract vi–vii

14. Ikuta K, Tono O, Oga M. Clinical outcome of microendoscopic posterior decompression for spinal stenosis associated with degenerative spondylolisthesis—minimum 2-year outcome of 37 patients. Minim Invasive Neurosurg 2008;51:267–271

15. Sasai K, Umeda M, Maruyama T, Wakabayashi E, Iida H. Microsurgical bilateral decompression via a unilateral approach for lumbar spinal canal stenosis including degenerative spondylolisthesis. J Neurosurg Spine 2008;9:554–559

16. Pao JL, Chen WC, Chen PQ. Clinical outcomes of microendoscopic decompressive laminotomy for degenerative lumbar spinal stenosis. Eur Spine J 2009;18:672–678

17. Palmer S, Turner R, Palmer R. Bilateral decompressive surgery in lumbar spinal stenosis associated with spondylolisthesis: unilateral approach and use of a microscope and tubular retractor system. Neurosurg Focus 2002;13:E4

18. Ogden AT, Bresnahan L, Smith JS, Natarajan R, Fessler RG. Biomechanical comparison of traditional and minimally invasive intradural tumor exposures using finite element analysis. Clin Biomech (Bristol, Avon) 2009;24:143–147

19. Jansson KA, Németh G, Granath F, Blomqvist P. Spinal stenosis re-operation rate in Sweden is 11% at 10 years—a national analysis of 9,664 operations. Eur Spine J 2005;14:659–663

20. Huang T-J, Hsu RW, Li YY, Cheng CC. Less systemic cytokine response in patients following microendoscopic versus open lumbar discectomy. J Orthop Res 2005;23:406–411

21. Kim KT, Lee SH, Suk KS, Bae SC. The quantitative analysis of tissue injury markers after mini-open lumbar fusion. Spine (Phila Pa 1976) 2006;31:712–716

22. Rosen DS, O'Toole JE, Eichholz KM, et al. Minimally invasive lumbar spinal decompression in the elderly: outcomes of 50 patients aged 75 years and older. Neurosurgery 2007;60:503–509

23. Rosen DS, Ferguson SD, Ogden AT, Huo D, Fessler RG. Obesity and self-reported outcome after minimally invasive lumbar spinal fusion surgery. Neurosurgery 2008;63:956–960

24. O'Toole JE, Eichholz KM, Fessler RG. Surgical site infection rates after minimally invasive spinal surgery. J Neurosurg Spine 2009;11:471–476

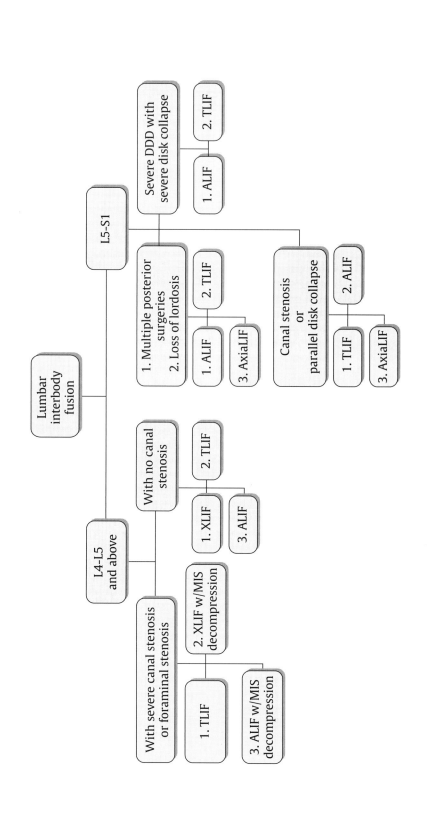

7

Minimally Invasive Transforaminal Lumbar Interbody Fusion

Vishal C. Gala and Regis W. Haid Jr.

Low back pain is among the most common reasons individuals seek medical attention in the United States.[1] Although the etiology of low back pain is multifactorial and most often managed with conservative, nonsurgical treatment, some patients require more intensive treatment in the form of surgery. Lumbar spinal fusion is sometimes employed in the treatment of degenerative conditions of the spine, such as facet arthropathy, degenerative disk disease, and spondylolisthesis, as well as in selected cases of spinal fractures, scoliosis, and tumors. Several studies over the past 2 decades have shown that the ability to achieve successful arthrodesis of spinal segments is enhanced by the use of instrumentation.[2] The use of spinal instrumentation, such as interbody spacers, pedicle screws and rods, and spinous process plates, has become widely accepted as the standard of care in lumbar spinal fusion surgery.

The use of spinal instrumentation has traditionally required wide and extensive exposure of the osseous anatomy of the lumbar spine to provide adequate exposure and visualization of anatomical landmarks. As a consequence, significant muscle dissection is required, resulting in denervation of the paraspinous musculature, bleeding, and retractor-induced muscle injury due to ischemia.[3-5] In addition, the dissection of the supporting ligamentous structures of the spine can often result in iatrogenic instability at adjacent levels.

Technological advancements in equipment and instrumentation, such as digital fluoroscopy, image guidance, high-resolution endoscopy, and microscopy, along with tubular dilators and working channels, have allowed for the development of minimally invasive surgical (MIS) techniques for the surgical treatment of degenerative spinal disorders. With the use of small portals of entry or working corridors, injury to the surrounding muscles and ligaments of the spine is minimized. Once appropriate access is obtained, the same surgical objectives of decompression of the neural elements and/or stabilization of the spine may be accomplished. Therefore, perhaps the term *minimal access* is a more accurate description. The array of modern MIS procedures for the spine are distinguished from previous "fad" procedures for the spine in that they are not limited to treating a single pathological process, nor are they based upon a single, heavily marketed device or technology. Rather, they are a concept that may be applied to several different clinical scenarios throughout the length of the spine.

With respect to the lumbar spine, the development of tubular retractor systems along with percutaneous pedicle screw systems has allowed for the application of minimally invasive techniques for conditions requiring fusion in the lumbar spine. This chapter describes the technique of minimally invasive transforaminal lumbar interbody fusion (MI-TLIF) along with the indications, decision-making process, and potential complications.

◆ Preoperative Evaluation

All patients should undergo a detailed and through history and physical examination. Radiologic evaluation must include either magnetic resonance imaging (MRI) or postmyelogram computed tomography (CT) to define the patient's specific pathoanatomy. Anteroposterior (AP), lateral, and dynamic flexion-extension plain radiographs are also critical to evaluate the patient for instability. Electromyography and nerve conduction studies may also provide supporting evidence to localize a patient's specific radiculopathy.

◆ Operative Technique

Patients are placed under general endotracheal anesthesia. A Foley catheter is placed. Use of an arterial line is discretionary based upon the patient's comorbidities. Sequential pneumatic compression devices are placed on the lower extremities. Leads are placed for somatosensory evoked potentials, and free run electromyography and baselines are obtained. Neurophysiological monitoring allows for continuous assessment of the integrity of the involved nerve roots and allows for the option of screw stimulation to ensure that the pedicle has not been breached during instrumentation.

The patient is placed in the prone position on a Jackson flat-top table outfitted with gel chest rolls. The flat-top table facilitates easy movement of the fluoroscopic C-arm during the operation. Gel rolls allow for maintenance of normal lordosis as opposed to a Wilson frame, which may place the patient in some degree of kyphosis or flat back. Prophylactic antibiotics are administered and standard surgical prep is performed. The surgeon is positioned on the side of the patient's most significant pathology. In cases of bilateral pathology, it is the surgeon's preference. The base of the fluoroscope is placed on the side opposite the surgeon.

With the assistance of AP fluoroscopy, the midline is marked. From there, a parallel line is drawn 4 to 4.5 cm laterally. A lateral image is obtained to localize the disk space of interest. In two-level cases, the incision is localized over the intervening vertebral body. Local anesthetic (0.25 to 0.5% bupivacaine) is injected into the skin, subcutaneous tissues, and musculature. The needle is also used to confirm the trajectory into the disk space. A small puncture incision is then made with a #11 blade. A Steinmann pin or K-wire is then advanced in a slightly medial trajectory toward the ipsilateral facet complex. Fluoroscopic guidance should be utilized during this process of docking and dilation to ensure that the spinal canal is not entered. Once confirmation is obtained by fluoroscopy that the K-wire is docked on the facet, the incision is lengthened symmetrically to match the diameter of the tubular retractor, typically 20 to 25 mm (depending on surgeon preference). The first dilator is then placed over the K-wire and the K-wire removed. Utilizing a rotatory motion, sequential dilators are then placed to split the musculature until the diameter of the tubular working channel is reached. Several different proprietary systems are available; some offer expandable blades as well. The working channel is then secured with a table-mounted flexible arm based on the side opposite the surgeon. At this point, the operation may proceed under loupe magnification with a headlight or with the assistance of an operating microscope.

The working channel should be docked over the facet of interest. It is paramount to carefully identify the midline spinous process and ipsilateral facet joint prior to any bone removal. With the oblique orientation of the tubular retractor, it is possible to inadvertently cross to the contralateral side of the spinal canal, especially in an obese patient. The facet should be visualized in the lateral half of the working channel, with the laminofacet junction and lateral portion of the lamina in the medial half of the working channel. Monopolar cautery is then used to dissect off any remaining soft tissue. The entirety of the working channel should be cleared of soft tissue to optimize visualization of the relatively small working corridor. The prominence of the top of the facet facilitates identification of the bony elements, and dissection should begin here to avoid entry into the spinal canal. The inferior edge of the superior lamina is then identified and the sublaminar plane developed with a curette. Utilizing curettes, rongeurs, and a high-speed drill, the surgeon performs a hemilaminotomy, extending rostrally to the superior pedicle and then caudally to the inferior lamina to the level of the inferior pedicle. A generous laminotomy and facetectomy must be performed to safely access the disk space and insert an interbody graft. Fluoroscopy should also be utilized to ensure that the pedicle is not entered with the drill.[6] The ligamentum is left in place to allow safer removal of the bone. To avoid potential dural injuries, all bony decompression should be performed prior to excision of the ligamentum flavum and exposure of the dura and neural elements. With a small working corridor and a narrow working angle, primary repair of a dural rent may be challenging but is possible with the use of microsurgical instruments. For small tears, onlay dural substitute may be placed over the durotomy and then a coat of fibrin glue or commercially available dural sealant placed over the synthetic pledget. Only in cases where persistent cerebrospinal fluid (CSF) leakage is observed after this maneuver is the option of a lumbar drain considered. Converting the procedure to an open one will typically serve to enlarge the area for a potential pseudomeningocele to form; therefore, it is best to maintain a smaller potential space. If the durotomy occurs prior to the interbody portion of the procedure, consideration may be given to proceeding with a posterolateral fusion alone.[7]

Bone fragments can be harvested for use as autograft. After bony decompression is completed, the subligamentous plane is developed and the ligamentum flavum excised. The disk space, lateral thecal sac, and traversing nerve root should be visualized, whereas the exiting nerve root may or may not be visualized depending upon the extent of bony removal. The thecal sac and nerve root should be gently retracted medially and all epidural veins over the disk space coagulated. If an adequate exposure has been obtained, minimal retraction is required. In rare instances of large exiting nerve roots or conjoined nerve roots that cover the disk space, interbody fusion may not be feasible. In these instances, consideration should be given to performing a posterolateral fusion alone.

The disk space is then incised and a thorough diskectomy performed with curettes and rongeurs. The end plates are then prepared with rotating cutters, rasps, and end plate scrapers. A series of dilators are then placed to distract the disk space and increase disk space height. Interbody grafting material is then placed. Typically this involves the placement of a sponge of recombinant human bone morphogenetic protein-2 (rhBMP-2) in combination with morcellized bone autograft into the ventral portion of the disk space. (The use of rhBMP-2 in this setting is an off-label use of the agent per the Food and Drug Administration.) An additional sponge of rhBMP-2 is placed within a polyether-ether-ketone (PEEK) cage (available in a variety of shapes and sizes). Synthetic PEEK most closely matches the modulus of elasticity of human bone, carries zero risk of disease transmission, and does not possess the problem of donor site morbidity or recipient rejection. Other options for interbody cages are also available: carbon fiber cages, machined allograft bone dowels, titanium cages, and absorbable spacers. Fluoroscopy is utilized to confirm appropriate interbody graft placement.

Contralateral pathology may be addressed indirectly on the basis of distraction of the intervertebral disk space, resulting in ligamentotaxis and an increase in the foraminal diameter. In cases of severe contralateral foraminal stenosis and central canal stenosis, the tubular working channel may be angled medially to decompress the central canal by undercutting the spinous process and contralateral hemilamina.

Attention is then turned to placement of pedicle screws. In cases where an expandable retractor has been used and a mini-open-type technique employed, ipsilateral pedicle screws are placed under direct visualization utilizing landmarks. In most MI-TLIF cases, the tubular retractor is withdrawn. Fluoroscopy is then utilized to place ipsilateral percutaneous pedicle screws through the existing incision utilizing K-wires and a cannulated screw system. Contralateral percutaneous screws are placed through small stab incisions in a similar fashion.

The standard technique for percutaneous screw placement involves fluoroscopic placement of a Jamshidi bone biopsy needle through the pedicle to access the vertebral body. One technique involves angling the fluoroscope to target the pedicle in a "bull's eye" fashion. The Jamshidi needle is placed into the center of the bull's eye and tapped several millimeters into the pedicle. A K-wire is then advanced through the Jamshidi 1 to 2 cm into the pedicle. An AP fluoroscopic image is the obtained to confirm center placement of all four K-wires. A lateral image is then obtained to assess the sagittal plane trajectory, and the K-wires are all advanced into the body. Cannulated drill-taps are then advanced over the K-wires. Cannulated screws with attached screw extenders are then placed and the K-wires removed.[8] Particular care should be taken when cannulated screws are used over

K-wires to ensure that the K-wires do not advance anteriorly through the vertebral body into the abdomen.[9] Intraoperative pedicle screw stimulation can be useful in assessing placement because it provides information as to the relative location of the pedicle screw in relation to the nerve root.[10] If an action potential is obtained at 10 mA or below, the screw should be removed and the screw path assessed for a cortical breach. Rods are passed and the locking screws affixed and given a final tightening. Several minimally invasive percutaneous pedicle screw–rod systems are available.

◆ Discussion

The transforaminal interbody fusion is a well-established technique for achieving circumferential fusion through a single, posterior approach.[11] The safety and efficacy of the open TLIF procedure are well established.[7,12–16] Fortunately, advances in imaging technology and instrumentation have allowed for the procedure to be performed using minimally invasive techniques.[17]

The basic indications for the MI-TLIF are identical to those for a traditional open lumbar fusion: spondylolisthesis with instability (grade I or II) and/or associated foraminal stenosis with radiculopathy (unilateral or bilateral), severe degenerative disk disease with mechanical low back pain, recurrent disk herniation with significant mechanical low back pain, third time or greater recurrent disk herniation with radiculopathy, and postlaminectomy kyphosis. Two-level TLIF may be performed through a single skin incision, although depending upon the levels and degree of lordosis, a more extensive fascial incision or a second dilation may be required. Patients requiring a fusion who have undergone a previous lumbar laminectomy for stenosis or multiple diskectomies are good candidates for an MI-TLIF because the paramedian approach through naive muscle avoids scar tissue and reduces the risks of nerve injury or a spinal fluid leak.

Obesity or morbid obesity is not a contraindication to minimally invasive spine surgery. Minimally invasive procedures may be routinely performed in obese patients. Indeed, several recent studies have found no difference in outcomes or complication rates between obese patients and nonobese patients who have undergone minimally invasive lumbar diskectomy/decompression or fusion.[18–21] Rosen et al recently reported a case series of 110 overweight or obese patients who underwent minimally invasive lumbar fusion and found that BMI had no significant relationship with self-reported outcome measures, operative time, length of hospital stay, or complications.[19] Obese patients are at increased risk for complications following spinal surgery, particularly surgical site infections, because larger incisions are required and larger cavities are created to access the deeper spine.[22–25] The use of a tubular retractor allows the surgeon to obtain exposure in the obese patient with the same size incision utilized in the nonobese patient. The obese patient then also experiences the same benefits as the nonobese patient from a minimal access approach. This patient population does pose a particular challenge with respect to placement of instrumentation in the MI-TLIF due to poor fluoroscopic visualization of anatomical landmarks and the limitations in tubular retractor length. This can be overcome with the use of longer tubular retractor systems generally used for direct or extreme lateral approaches. Certainly, working with tubular retractors that are greater than 8 cm in length can be difficult, with some challenges posed with respect to lighting, visualization, and manipulation of the retractor in many planes of motion.

Relative contraindications for the MI-TLIF include multilevel procedures (greater than two interspaces) and severe osteoporosis (higher risk of graft subsidence and instrumentation failure). The MI-TLIF is contraindicated in cases of significant scoliosis, high-grade spondylolisthesis, or gross spinal instability from trauma.[26] In cases of scoliosis, the trajectory of tube placement and pedicle screw placement is difficult to ascertain with standard fluoroscopy. Reduction of high-grade spondylolisthesis or of gross, traumatic instability, similarly, is best accomplished through an open technique because it affords the greatest degree of access for realignment and stabilization.

Interestingly, minimally invasive approaches may be of little or no benefit in very thin patients with limited subcutaneous fat, specifically those with a skin to facet joint distance of less than 4 cm. In this patient population, the degree of muscle dissection required for tube placement and exposure of the bony elements may result in more soft tissue injury than a standard subperiosteal dissection performed through a midline incision.

Initial cadaveric feasibility studies of the MI-TLIF procedure were performed by Fessler and colleagues in 2002. They demonstrated that the procedure could be performed safely and effectively.[27] This was followed by an initial case-control study in 2005 that reported a significant decrease in intraoperative blood loss, postoperative narcotic use, and hospital length of stay in patients who underwent an MI-TLIF versus patients who underwent an open lumbar fusion.[28]

Park and Foley reported a series of 40 patients with a minimum 2-year follow-up (mean of 35 months) in patients with spondylolisthesis who underwent MI-TLIF. Thirty of the 40 patients had degenerative spondylolisthesis, whereas 10 had a congenital spondylolysis.[29] They achieved on average a 76% reduction in anterior translation with statistically significant postoperative declines in visual analog pain scores for back and leg pain and in the Oswestry Disability Index. These results compare favorably with open procedures for the same indication.

A German series of 43 patients reported a case-control study comparing MI-TLIF to open TLIF. They found that patients who underwent MI-TLIF had similar operative times and fusion rates but statistically significant reductions in blood loss and postoperative pain. No difference in clinical outcomes was seen at 8 and 16 months utilizing standardized functional questionnaires.[30]

Another case-control study with 2-year follow-up comparing open TLIF to MI-TLIF found statistically significant reductions in blood loss, postoperative narcotic use, and hospital length of stay in patients who underwent MI-TLIF.[31] Fusion rates were comparable in the two groups. Both groups achieved statistically significant improvements in Oswestry Disability Index, visual analog scores for back and lower limb pain, and quality of life (SF-36 scores).

An Australian prospective study of 47 patients with spondylolisthesis comparing minimally invasive lumbar fusion and open lumbar fusion found equivalent outcomes with respect to improvement in back and leg pain, reduction of spondylolisthesis, and rates of fusion. The minimally invasive group, however, were ambulatory sooner, achieved independent mobilization sooner, and had a shorter length of hospital stay (4 days vs 7 days).[32]

◆ Conclusion

In experienced hands, the MI-TLIF may be performed safely, effectively, and with the benefits of decreased blood loss, reduced postoperative narcotic use, and decreased length of hospital stay. When compared with other interbody fusion techniques, such as anterior lumbar interbody fusion or extreme lateral interbody fusion, the MI-TLIF is the most appropriate choice in patients with severe canal stenosis. This approach may be superior in the obese population when compared with the traditional subperiosteal exposure due to the decreased incision size and tissue dissection that the use of tubular retractors affords. Patients with previous surgeries may also benefit from the paramedian trajectory through naive tissue. Severe scoliosis and high-grade spondylolistheses are relative contraindications.

Case Illustration

A 55-year-old female presented with a history of progressive low back and bilateral lower extremity pain and numbness. She had undergone extensive conservative treatment but failed to obtain sustained relief of her symptoms. MRI revealed a mobile L5–S1 grade 2 spondylolisthesis with bilateral neuroforaminal stenosis. She underwent an L5–S1 MI-TLIF with placement of percutaneous pedicle screws (**Figs. 7.1A,B, 7.2, 7.3, 7.4,** and **7.5**). She had resolution of her back and leg pain following surgery and demonstrated stable fusion on 1-year x-rays.

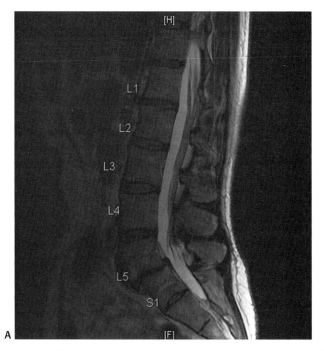

Fig. 7.1 (A) Sagittal magnetic resonance imaging scan demonstrating L5–S1 spondylolisthesis. (*continued*)

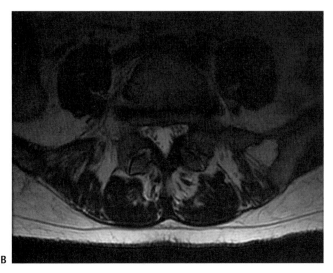

Fig. 7.1 (*continued*) (B) Axial magnetic resonance imaging scan demonstrating L5–S1 spondylolisthesis.

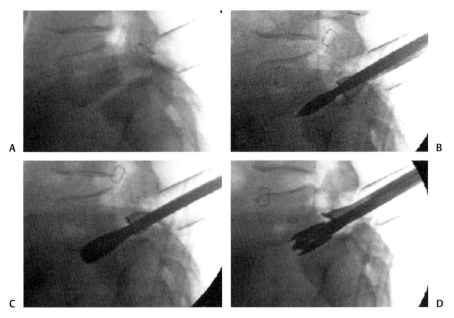

Fig. 7.2 (A–D) Intraoperative fluoroscopic images illustrating tube placement, facetectomy, and diskectomy.

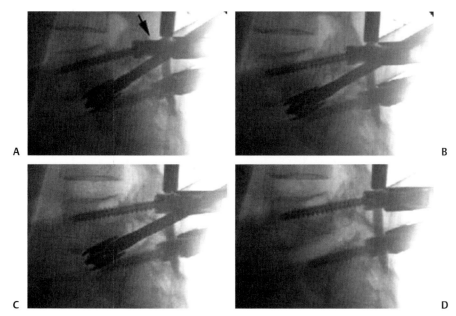

A   B

C   D

Fig. 7.3 **(A–D)** Intraoperative fluoroscopic images demonstrating reduction of spondylolisthesis after contralateral percutaneous pedicle screw placement and distraction across the interspace.

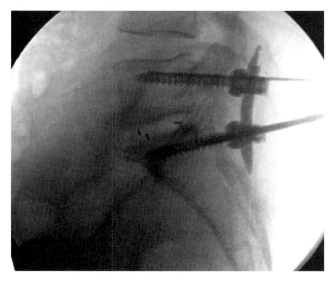

Fig. 7.4 Final fluoroscopic image after reduction, placement of the interbody graft and rod insertion.

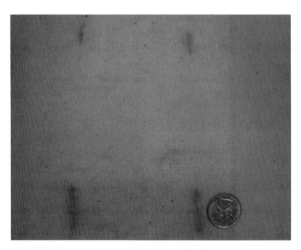

Fig. 7.5 Incisions required for single-level minimally invasive transforaminal lumbar interbody fusion.

References

1. Manek NJ, MacGregor AJ. Epidemiology of back disorders: prevalence, risk factors, and prognosis. Curr Opin Rheumatol 2005;17:134–140

2. Zdeblick TA. A prospective, randomized study of lumbar fusion: preliminary results. Spine (Phila Pa 1976) 1993;18:983–991

3. Kawaguchi Y, Matsui H, Tsuji H. Back muscle injury after posterior lumbar spine surgery: a histologic and enzymatic analysis. Spine (Phila Pa 1976) 1996;21:941–944

4. Kawaguchi Y, Matsui H, Tsuji H. Back muscle injury after posterior lumbar spine surgery, II: Histologic and histochemical analyses in humans. Spine (Phila Pa 1976) 1994;19:2598–2602

5. See DH, Kraft GH. Electromyography in paraspinal muscles following surgery for root compression. Arch Phys Med Rehabil 1975;56:80–83

6. Mimran R, Perez-Curet M, Fessler R, Jacob R. Endoscopic lumbar laminectomy for stenosis. In: Fessler R, ed. An Anatomic Approach to Minimally Invasive Spine Surgery. St. Louis, MO: Quality Medical Publishing; 2006:569–582

7. Rosenberg WS, Mummaneni PV. Transforaminal lumbar interbody fusion: technique, complications, and early results. Neurosurgery 2001;48:569–574

8. Isaacs RE, Podichetty VK, Sandhu FA, et al. Microendoscopically assisted transforaminal lumbar interbody fusion. In: Fessler R, Sekhar L, eds. Atlas of Neurosurgical Techniques: Spine and Peripheral Nerves. New York: Thieme; 2006:859–865

9. Perez-Cruet M. Percutaneous pedicle screw placement for spinal instrumentation. In: Perez-Cruet M, Khoo L, Fessler R, eds. An Anatomic Approach to Minimally Invasive Spine Surgery. St. Louis, MO: Quality Medical Publishing; 2006:583–590

10. Roedel A, Zak S, Fessler R. Pedicle screw stimulation in minimally invasive spinal instrumentation. In: Thirteenth Annual Meeting of the American Society of Neurophysiological Monitoring; Lake Buena Vista, FL; 2002

11. Harms J, Rolinger H. A one-stage procedure in operative treatment of spondylolistheses: dorsal traction-reposition and anterior fusion (author's transl) [in German]. Z Orthop Ihre Grenzgeb 1982;120:343–347

12. Humphreys SC, Hodges SD, Patwardhan AG, Eck JC, Murphy RB, Covington LA. Comparison of posterior and transforaminal approaches to lumbar interbody fusion. Spine (Phila Pa 1976) 2001; 26:567–571

13. Kwon BK, Berta S, Daffner SD, et al. Radiographic analysis of transforaminal lumbar interbody fusion for the treatment of adult isthmic spondylolisthesis. J Spinal Disord Tech 2003;16:469–476

14. Mummaneni PV, Haid RW, Rodts GE. Lumbar interbody fusion: state-of-the-art technical advances: invited submission from the Joint Section Meeting on Disorders of the Spine and Peripheral Nerves, March 2004. J Neurosurg Spine 2004;1:24–30

15. Mummaneni PV, Pan J, Haid RW, Rodts GE. Contribution of recombinant human bone morphogenetic protein-2 to the rapid creation of interbody fusion when used in transforaminal lumbar interbody fusion: a preliminary report. Invited submission from the Joint Section Meeting on Disorders of the Spine and Peripheral Nerves, March 2004. J Neurosurg Spine 2004;1:19–23

16. Salehi SA, Tawk R, Ganju A, LaMarca F, Liu JC, Ondra SL. Transforaminal lumbar interbody fusion: surgical technique and results in 24 patients. Neurosurgery 2004;54:368–374

17. Foley KT, Holly LT, Schwender JD. Minimally invasive lumbar fusion. Spine (Phila Pa 1976) 2003;28(15, Suppl):S26–S35

18. Tomasino A, Parikh K, Steinberger J, Knopman J, Boockvar J, Härtl R. Tubular microsurgery for lumbar discectomies and laminectomies in obese patients: operative results and outcome. Spine (Phila Pa 1976) 2009;34:E664–E672

19. Rosen DS, Ferguson SD, Ogden AT, Huo D, Fessler RG. Obesity and self-reported outcome after minimally invasive lumbar spinal fusion surgery. Neurosurgery 2008;63:956–960

20. Park P, Upadhyaya C, Garton HJ, Foley KT. The impact of minimally invasive spine surgery on perioperative complications in overweight or obese patients. Neurosurgery 2008;62:693–699

21. Cole JS IV, Jackson TR IV. Minimally invasive lumbar discectomy in obese patients. Neurosurgery 2007;61:539–544

22. Olsen MA, Mayfield J, Lauryssen C, et al. Risk factors for surgical site infection in spinal surgery. J Neurosurg 2003;98(2, Suppl):149–155

23. Patel N, Bagan B, Vadera S, et al. Obesity and spine surgery: relation to perioperative complications. J Neurosurg Spine 2007;6:291–297

24. Telfeian AE, Reiter GT, Durham SR, Marcotte P. Spine surgery in morbidly obese patients. J Neurosurg 2002;97(1, Suppl):20–24

25. Wimmer C, Gluch H, Franzreb M, Ogon M. Predisposing factors for infection in spine surgery: a survey of 850 spinal procedures. J Spinal Disord 1998;11:124–128

26. Mummaneni P, Lu D, Chi J. Minimally incisional transforaminal interbody fusion. In: Resnick D, Haid R, Wang J, eds. Surgical Management of Low Back Pain. New York: Thieme; 2009:110–116

27. Khoo LT, Palmer S, Laich DT, Fessler RG. Minimally invasive percutaneous posterior lumbar interbody fusion. Neurosurgery 2002;51(5, Suppl 2):S166–S181

28. Isaacs RE, Podichetty VK, Santiago P, et al. Minimally invasive microendoscopy-assisted transforaminal lumbar interbody fusion with instrumentation. J Neurosurg Spine 2005;3:98–105

29. Park P, Foley KT. Minimally invasive transforaminal lumbar interbody fusion with reduction of spondylolisthesis: technique and outcomes after a minimum of 2 years' follow-up. Neurosurg Focus 2008;25:E16

30. Scheufler KM, Dohmen H, Vougioukas VI. Percutaneous transforaminal lumbar interbody fusion for the treatment of degenerative lumbar instability. Neurosurgery 2007;60(4, Suppl 2):203–212

31. Peng CW, Yue WM, Poh SY, Yeo W, Tan SB. Clinical and radiological outcomes of minimally invasive versus open transforaminal lumbar interbody fusion. Spine (Phila Pa 1976) 2009;34:1385–1389

32. Ghahreman A, Ferch RD, Rao PJ, Bogduk N. Minimal access versus open posterior lumbar interbody fusion in the treatment of spondylolisthesis. Neurosurgery 2010;66:296–304

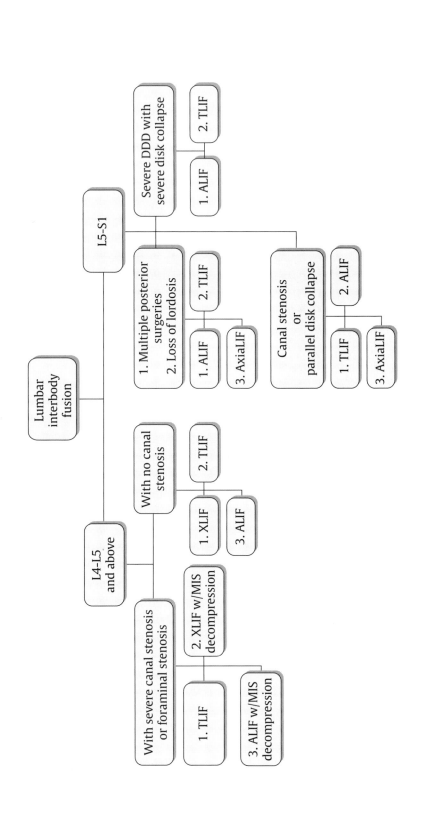

8

Alternative Approaches for Lumbar Fusion: eXtreme Lateral Interbody Fusion (XLIF)

Luiz H. M. Pimenta, Etevaldo Coutinho, and Leonardo Oliveira

Chronic low back pain has been recognized as a complex disorder associated with wide-ranging adverse consequences.[1-6] Patients suffering from a painful lumbar motion segment not resolved with conservative management gain benefit from lumbar arthrodesis.[7]

Lumbar spine fusion has become a commonly performed surgery, and its use continues to rise, with the annual number of spinal fusion operations increasing every year.[8] Initially, reconstructive spinal fusion surgery was used for the management of infectious conditions, adolescent scoliosis, and trauma. The indications for spinal fusion among these patients have remained largely unchanged. Based on these experiences, the use of spinal arthrodesis has been extended to treat degenerative lumbar disorders, spondylolisthesis, and disk-related problems.[9]

Anterior lumbar interbody fusion (ALIF) is the technique commonly used to achieve lumbar interbody arthrodesis. The ALIF allows restoration of disk space, lumbar lordosis, and spinal alignment, without compromising posterior tension bands.[10-13] Besides, resection of the disk eliminates a source of diskogenic back pain. Disadvantages of ALIF include the necessity of an access surgeon, high incidence of vascular injury, and retrograde ejaculation. In addition, ALIF is associated with increased operating time and blood loss, as well as prolonged recovery time.[14]

Minimally invasive surgical techniques have been demonstrated to provide several benefits, which include less tissue trauma, preservation of normal anatomical structures, and a faster recuperative period.[15-18]

The eXtreme Lateral Interbody Fusion (XLIF, NuVasive, Inc., San Diego, CA) approach may offer various clinical advantages over more traditional techniques for lumbar fusion.[19] This minimally invasive procedure realigns the end plates to a horizontal position through bilateral annular release, placement of a large implant across the disk space spanning the ring apophysis, and the effects of ligamentotaxis. The XLIF technique restores disk and foraminal heights, indirectly decompressing the neural elements, and promotes stabilization through an anterior intervertebral fusion.

◆ Preoperative Evaluation

Indications

Indications for the XLIF technique are the same as those for any interbody fusion, with the limitation of access only at disk levels above L5. Such patients typically suffer diskogenic pain due to segmental instability, disk degeneration, degenerative scoliosis, and/or grade 1 or 2 spondylolisthesis.[20-24] It may also be applied to patients who have failed prior surgery and require interbody fusion, or in cases of adjacent-level disease. Pseudarthrosis and failed lumbar total disk replacements have also been treated using the XLIF approach for retrieval and revision.

The XLIF approach has been successfully accomplished for levels above and including L4–5. Approaching the L5–S1 level using this technique is not recommended because of the risk of iliac vessel injury as well as the difficulty of accessing the disk space due to the iliac crest. For the L5–S1 level it is preferable to use a mini–open retroperitoneal approach or minimally invasive posterior approach.

Preoperative Imaging

Usually the initial x-ray workup begins with flexion and extension films to determine the amount of sagittal instability and the amount of kyphosis flexibility. Oblique views can be useful in this technique as well. A focused lumbar or thoracic view is helpful to evaluate disk height, disk asymmetry, and lateral listhesis.

Computed tomographic (CT) scans associated with myelographic study are used to evaluate central and foraminal stenosis. Magnetic resonance imaging (MRI) is useful for evaluating disk degeneration and foraminal stenosis. Other ancillary tests, such as diskography and facet blocks, are done to elucidate which levels should be included in the fusion procedure.

◆ Operative Technique

Patient Positioning

For the XLIF approach, the patient is placed and taped in a true 90 degree lateral decubitus position (**Fig. 8.1A**). A cross-table anteroposterior (AP) image helps to confirm the true 90 degree position. The table and/or patient should be flexed in such a way as to increase the distance between the iliac crest and the rib cage, especially useful at upper lumbar levels and at L4–5.

Incision

After aseptic treatment of the skin, a K-wire and lateral fluoroscopic image are used to identify the midposition of the disk of interest (**Fig. 8.2**). A mark is made on the

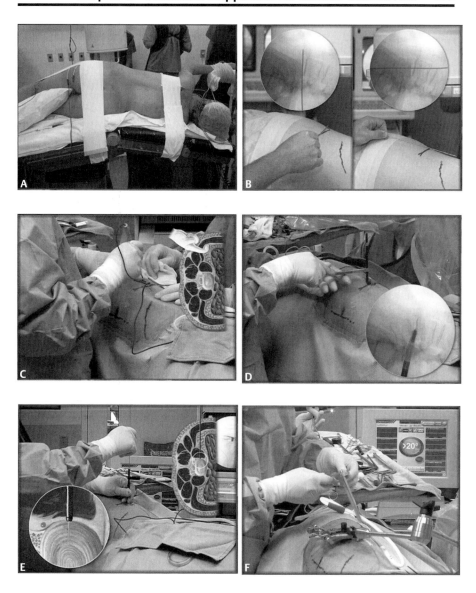

Fig. 8.1 eXtreme Lateral Interbody and Fusion (XLIF) surgical technique (NuVasive, Inc., San Diego, CA). **(A)** Patient positioning. **(B)** Index level identification. **(C)** Retroperitoneal access. **(D,E)**. Transpsoas access. **(F)** MaXcess tractor (NuVasive, Inc., San Diego, CA) insertion. (*continued*)

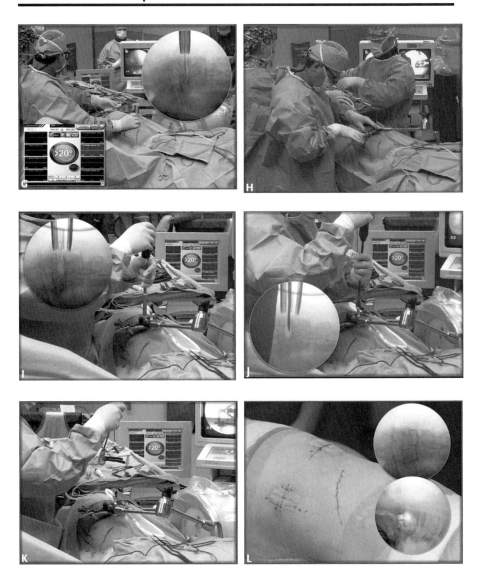

Fig. 8.1 (*continued*)   **(G)** NeuroVision Electromyographic System (NuVasive, Inc., San Diego, CA). **(H)** MaXcess fixation. **(I)** Diskectomy. **(J)** End plate preparation. **(K)** Implant insertion. **(L)** Surgical wounds.

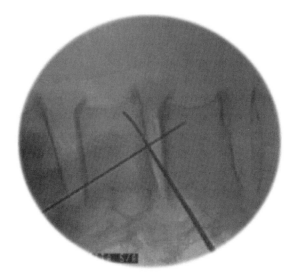

Fig. 8.2   K-wire and lateral fluoroscopy are used to identify the midposition of the disk.

patient's lateral side, overlying the center of the affected disk space (**Fig. 8.1B**); a small incision will be created for insertion of atraumatic tissue dilators and an expandable retractor (MaXcess, NuVasive, Inc., San Diego, CA), which will be the working portal (**Fig. 8.1C**). An incision posterior to this lateral marking is first made to introduce a finger into the retroperitoneal space to sweep open the space and ensure that any lateral attachments of the peritoneum are released to provide safe lateral entry.

Transpsoas Access

With the retroperitoneal space identified, the finger is brought up under the lateral skin marking and an incision is made at this direct lateral location for the introduction of an initial dilator. The finger in the retroperitoneal space is used to escort the dilator safely from the direct lateral incision to the psoas muscle, protecting the intra-abdominal contents. The dilator is then placed over the surface of the psoas muscle, exactly over the disk space to be operated, as confirmed by AP and lateral fluoroscopy (**Fig. 8.1D,E**). The fibers of the psoas muscle are then gently separated with the initial dilator using blunt dissection and the NeuroVision electromyographic (EMG) monitoring system (NuVasive, Inc.) to assess proximity of the lumbar nerve roots to the advancing dilator. The dilation continues with the surgeon delicately spreading the midportion of the psoas muscle fibers while avoiding the nerves of the lumbar plexus, until the lateral surface of the disk is reached. An expandable retractor (MaXcess) is advanced over the last dilator, also under NeuroVision guidance, locked to the surgical table, and expanded to expose the lateral disk space (**Fig. 8.1F–H**).

Under direct illuminated vision, a thorough diskectomy is performed using standard instruments. The posterior annulus is left intact, with the annulotomy window centered in the anterior half of the disk space and wide enough to accommodate a large implant. Disk removal and release of the contralateral annulus using a Cobb elevator provides the opportunity to place a long implant that will rest on both lateral margins of the apophyseal ring, maximizing end plate support (**Fig. 8.1I,J**). Interbody distraction and implant placement in this anterior and bilateral apophyseal position provide strong support for disk height restoration and sagittal and coronal plane imbalance correction (**Fig. 8.1K**).

Closure

The exposure is copiously irrigated, and the retractor is removed slowly so as to observe the psoas muscle rebounding and to confirm hemostasis. The incisions are closed with standard material (**Fig. 8.1L**). No drains have thus far been required.

Complications and Management

There is no surgery without possible complications, including those due to anesthesia, iatrogenic injury, or preexisting conditions. In comparison, our results demonstrate a lower level of complications due to the minimally invasive nature of the procedure. We observed minor complications in the immediate postoperative period, such as tenderness with hip flexion on the operative side and, less commonly, sensory disturbance in the operative side leg. Painful dysesthesias and motor disturbance are rare, but possible. In these cases, a CT scan is recommended to rule out a psoas hematoma. If a hematoma is found, draining it should improve symptoms.

◆ Discussion

The XLIF technique is a modification of the retroperitoneal approach to the lumbar spine. The technique was first presented in 2001 by Pimenta, who had performed more than 100 lateral transpsoas surgeries between 1998 and 2000.[19]

When compared with anterior laparoscopic approaches to the lumbar spine, the lateral approach has several advantages. First, a general surgeon is not needed for access. A far lateral approach eliminates the need to violate or retract the peritoneum, or to retract the great vessels. Second, a far lateral approach avoids many of the known complications of laparoscopic anterior approaches, such as damage to the great vessels during mobilization,[25,26] and retrograde ejaculation,[27,28] most likely from disturbance of the superior hypogastric nerve plexus. Third, the most significant advantage we report between the laparoscopic ALIF and our XLIF is in operative time. When compared with mini–open laparotomy, a laparoscopic ALIF has been noted to have longer operative time.[29]

Limitations do exist with this far lateral approach. Dissecting the psoas major must be done carefully so as not to injure the nerves of the lumbar plexus or cause significant trauma to the muscle. Prior reports of lateral retroperitoneal approaches included mobilization of the psoas muscle from the lumbar spine, but a high incidence of transient numbness along the genitofemoral nerve has been reported after retraction of the psoas muscle.[30,31] Because the XLIF approach requires neither retraction of the psoas major nor significant dilation of the dissection site in the muscle, transient sensory deficits along the genitofemoral nerve are unlikely. Use of the NeuroVision EMG monitoring system is critical to the safe passage by the nerves within the psoas muscle itself.

As with most minimally disruptive spinal techniques, intraoperative fluoroscopy use is critical. The surgical results of this procedure have shown that it is a safe and reproducible technique, with quick recovery and improvements in pain and function scales. Disk heights were restored and stability maintained by preserving ligamentous structures and inserting a large interbody implant. This indirectly improves the foraminal area and results in reduction of radiculopathy. Sagittal balance was maintained or improved by placement of the implant in an anterior position (**Fig. 8.3**). Coronal imbalances were corrected by ensuring full bilateral end plate coverage by the implant. Our patients have shown solid fusion progression, apparently uncompromised by the technique.

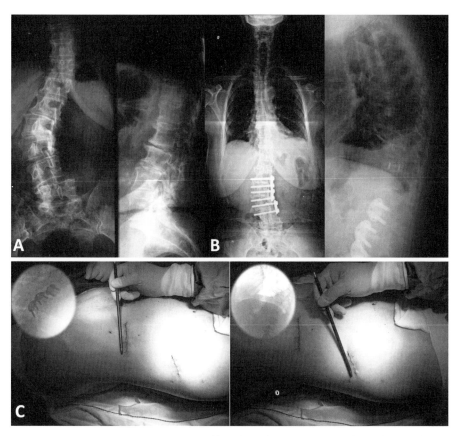

Fig. 8.3   Patient example. **(A)** A 62-year-old female with degenerative scoliosis, back and right leg pain, neurogenic claudication, and inability to walk more than 100 m. **(B)** One week after surgery, we can see improvement of the coronal balance using eXtreme Lateral Interbody Fusion (XLIF, NuVasive, Inc., San Diego, CA). **(C)** Seven-level surgery achieved with two small incisions.

◆ Conclusion

The XLIF approach is highly recommended for lumbar fusion. It is a feasible, safe, and effective technique. The complication rate has been lower than that with traditional surgical methods of treatment. Subsidence is the most common complication in the XLIF stand-alone technique, but our experience has shown no clinical compromise in the final result. We have been successfully performing fusion using stand-alone cages through a lateral minimally invasive approach (**Fig. 8.4**), decreasing pain, indirectly decompressing neurological structures, restoring disk height, and stopping the curve progression, in cases of degenerative scoliosis.

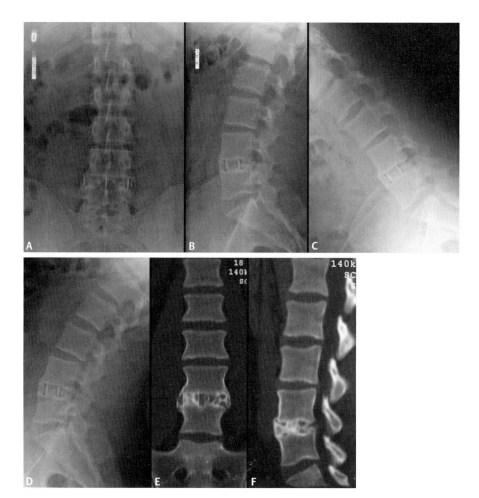

Fig. 8.4   Case illustration. **(A)** Anterioposterior, **(B)** lateral, **(C)** flexion, **(D)** extension, and **(E,F)** computed tomographic scans showing solid fusion 12 months after the eXtreme Lateral Interbody Fusion (XLIF, NuVasive, Inc., San Diego, CA) stand-alone procedure.

References

1. Weiner DK, Sakamoto S, Perera S, Breuer P. Chronic low back pain in older adults: prevalence, reliability, and validity of physical examination findings. J Am Geriatr Soc 2006;54:11–20

2. Lavsky-Shulan M, Wallace RB, Kohout FJ, Lemke JH, Morris MC, Smith IM. Prevalence and functional correlates of low back pain in the elderly: the Iowa 65+ Rural Health Study. J Am Geriatr Soc 1985;33:23–28

3. Reid MC, Williams CS, Concato J, Tinetti ME, Gill TM. Depressive symptoms as a risk factor for disabling back pain in community-dwelling older persons. J Am Geriatr Soc 2003;51:1710–1717

4. Gentili A, Weiner DK, Kuchibhatil M, Edinger JD. Factors that disturb sleep in nursing home residents. Aging (Milano) 1997;9:207–213

5. Carey TS, Evans A, Hadler N, Kalsbeek W, McLaughlin C, Fryer J. Care-seeking among individuals with chronic low back pain. Spine (Phila Pa 1976) 1995;20:312–317

6. Bosley BN, Weiner DK, Rudy TE, Granieri E. Is chronic nonmalignant pain associated with decreased appetite in older adults? Preliminary evidence. J Am Geriatr Soc 2004;52:247–251

7. Benz RJ, Garfin SR. Current techniques of decompression of the lumbar spine. Clin Orthop Relat Res 2001;(384):75–81

8. Tanaka N, An HS, Lim TH, Fujiwara A, Jeon CH, Haughton VM. The relationship between disc degeneration and flexibility of the lumbar spine. Spine J 2001;1:47–56

9. Aryan HE, Lu DC, Acosta FL Jr, Ames CP. Stand-alone anterior lumbar discectomy and fusion with plate: initial experience. Surg Neurol 2007;68:7–13

10. Crock HV. Anterior lumbar interbody fusion: indications for its use and notes on surgical technique. Clin Orthop Relat Res 1982;165:157–163

11. Lund T, Oxland TR, Jost B, et al. Interbody cage stabilization in the lumbar spine: biomechanical evaluation of cage design, posterior instrumentation and bone density. J Bone Joint Surg Br 1998;80:351–359

12. Madan SS, Harley JM, Boeree NR. Anterior lumbar interbody fusion: does stable anterior fixation matter? Eur Spine J 2003;12:386–392

13. Resnick DK, Choudhri TF, Dailey AT, et al; American Association of Neurological Surgeons/Congress of Neurological Surgeons. Guidelines for the performance of fusion procedures for degenerative disease of the lumbar spine, XI: Interbody techniques for lumbar fusion. J Neurosurg Spine 2005;2:692–699

14. Rajaraman V, Vingan R, Roth P, Heary RF, Conklin L, Jacobs GB. Visceral and vascular complications resulting from anterior lumbar interbody fusion. J Neurosurg 1999;91(1, Suppl):60–64

15. Dewald CJ, Millikan KW, Hammerberg KW, Doolas A, Dewald RL. An open, minimally invasive approach to the lumbar spine. Am Surg 1999;65:61–68

16. Foley KT, Holly LT, Schwender JD. Minimally invasive lumbar fusion. Spine (Phila Pa 1976) 2003;28(15, Suppl):S26–S35

17. German JW, Foley KT. Minimal access surgical techniques in the management of the painful lumbar motion segment. Spine (Phila Pa 1976) 2005;30(16, Suppl):S52–S59

18. Lin RM, Huang KY, Lai KA. Mini-open anterior spine surgery for anterior lumbar diseases. Eur Spine J 2008;17:691–697

19. Ozgur BM, Aryan HE, Pimenta L, Taylor WR. Extreme Lateral Interbody Fusion (XLIF): a novel surgical technique for anterior lumbar interbody fusion. Spine J 2006;6:435–443

20. Fessler RG. Minimally invasive spine surgery. Neurosurgery 2002;51(5, Suppl):Siii–iv

21. Hovorka I, de Peretti F, Damon F, Arcamone H, Argenson C. Five years' experience of the retroperitoneal lumbar and thoracolumbar surgery. Eur Spine J 2000;9(1, Suppl 1):S30–S34

22. Iwahara T, Ikeda K, Hirabayashi K. Results of anterior spine fusion by extraperitoneal approach for spondylolisthesis. Nippon Seikeigeka Gakkai Zasshi 1963;36:1049–1067

23. Lane LD, Moore SE. Transperitoneal approach to intervertebral disc in the lumbar area. Ann Surg 1948;127:537–551

24. Madan SS, Boeree NR. Comparison of instrumented anterior interbody fusion with instrumented circumferential lumbar fusion. Eur Spine J 2003;12:567–575

25. Baker JK, Reardon PR, Reardon MJ, Heggeness MH. Vascular injury in anterior lumbar surgery. Spine (Phila Pa 1976) 1993;18:2227–2230

26. Regan JJ, McAfee PC, Guyer RD, Aronoff RJ. Laparoscopic fusion of the lumbar spine in a multicenter series of the first 34 consecutive patients. Surg Laparosc Endosc 1996;6:459–468

27. Christensen FB, Bünger CE. Retrograde ejaculation after retroperitoneal lower lumbar interbody fusion. Int Orthop 1997;21:176–180

28. Flynn JC, Price CT. Sexual complications of anterior fusion of the lumbar spine. Spine (Phila Pa 1976) 1984;9:489–492

29. Liu JC, Ondra SL, Angelos P, Ganju A, Landers ML. Is laparoscopic anterior lumbar interbody fusion a useful minimally invasive procedure? Neurosurgery 2002;51(5, Suppl):S155–S158

30. Bergey DL, Villavicencio AT, Goldstein T, Regan JJ. Endoscopic lateral transpsoas approach to the lumbar spine. Spine (Phila Pa 1976) 2004;29:1681–1688

31. Nakamura H, Ishikawa T, Konishi S, Seki M, Yamano Y. Psoas strapping technique: a new technique for laparoscopic anterior lumbar interbody fusion. J Am Coll Surg 2000;191:686–688

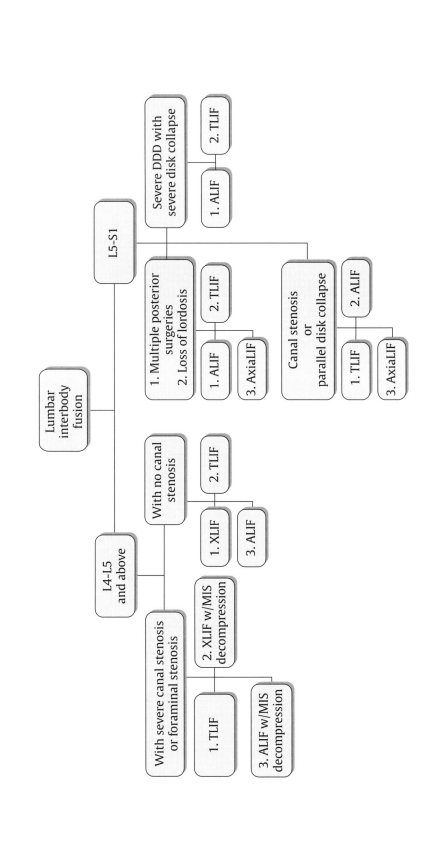

9

Alternative Approaches for Lumbar Fusion: Axial Lumbar Interbody Fusion (AxiaLIF)

Pierce D. Nunley

Minimally invasive lumbar spine surgery has moved from the feasibility stage in recent years to being achievable due to the development of safe and reproducible advanced access technology and approaches to the lumbar spine. Many innovative surgeons have driven this development by their desire to reduce the iatrogenic morbidity while expediting and improving the fusion and functional outcomes of traditional open spine surgery. On occasion, this can further be expanded to allow the surgeon to treat pathology that before would not have been safe or efficacious to treat.

The disadvantages of open lumbar surgery include the need for excessive muscle dissection, nerve retraction, ligamentous and bony dissection, vascular exposure, and disruption of the annulus fibrosus, anterior longitudinal ligament (ALL), and posterior longitudinal ligament (PLL). Traditional fusion approaches can produce undesirable scarring and destabilization of the native anatomy solely related to the exposure. All minimally invasive surgery (MIS) techniques seek to minimize or eliminate these disadvantages.

The aim of axial stabilization, using over-the-wire percutaneous techniques, is to provide a similar diskectomy and end plate preparation and to implant an inherently stable fusion construct through smaller incisions and ports. The small axial working channel can make previously open maneuvers, such as access, diskectomy, and implant insertion, more reproducible regardless of the patient's body habitus.

For most MIS techniques, the approach mimics those commonly used in open approaches to the spine, that is, anterolateral, lateral, posterolateral, and extraforaminal exposure of the disk space and incision or excision of the annulus via tubular or expandable retractors.

When fusion and stabilization of the lumbosacral spine are indicated, an axial construct that spares the annulus and supporting tissues may offer significant advantages over other MIS techniques. The axial lumbar interbody fusion (AxiaLIF) system and technique (TranS1, Wilmington, NC) was developed to capitalize on the advantages of minimally invasive axial access and instrumentation in the least invasive manner. The technique represents a cohesion of established spinal reconstruction concepts and percutaneous access, image guidance, and advanced biomechanical implant technology.

Axial implants and constructs have been used previously in open spine surgery for high-grade slips and corpectomy. The parasagittal fibular strut and vertebral body replacement devices all used this principle.[1] A disadvantage of these constructs, however, is the need for open surgery to implant them in patients with degenerative disk disease with or without radiculopathy, including low-grade instability. The approach described here combines the inherent advantages of an axial stabilization and fusion with the least invasive access approach.

The spine is a well protected axial column with orthogonal axes defining the sagittal bending, coronal (lateral) bending, and torsional movements. The lumbar spine is surrounded by the viscera anteriorly and the paraspinal musculature, ligaments, and neural elements laterally and posteriorly. The employment of an axial approach avoids these key structures and allows for the design of unique constructs that can achieve the same standard-of-care arthrodesis principles that correspond with currently accepted surgical approaches and biomechanical constructs.

An axial approach to the anterior lumbar spine has the potential to improve the biomechanical performance of both fusion and motion-preservation constructs. With this access, posterior instrumentation, and proper technique, a robust axial construct can be placed to restore disk height, sagittal balance, and lordosis with minimal dissection and postoperative pain. Axial disk space entry can simplify the technique of end plate preparation for fusion by reducing the challenges of accessing a collapsed disk space.

This muscle-, annulus-, ALL-, and PLL-sparing approach, combined with a completely competent annulus to achieve ligamentum taxis, is another significant potential advantage of the axial technique that may be important in the successful evolution of motion-preserving implants.

Before its initial human application, the technique was tested and validated in both cadavers and porcine models. In a series of six porcine models and 15 cadavers, the instruments and technique for percutaneous axial lumbar interbody fusion (AxiaLIF) were developed. Successful axial access to the lumbar spine was achieved in all cases. The instruments evolved to permit fluoroscopically guided access, diskectomy, and stabilization of the L5–S1 motion segment through a single 2 cm incision.

In a small access feasibility series of three consecutive patients, biopsy of the lumbosacral disk and vertebral body region was performed for suspected pathological lesions by Cragg et al in May 2002.[2] The technique was used with no adverse events. Patients tolerated the procedure well with no significant postoperative pain or morbidity. In the following year a series of three patients underwent an arthrodesis procedure using the axial approach and were observed for 6 months with promising results.[2] A human pilot study was initiated with Pimenta et al in November 2003 that included 35 patients with very promising results.[3]

The first AxiaLIF was performed by Levy (University of Buffalo)[4] in January 2005 after U.S. Food and Drug Administration (FDA) regulatory clearance was obtained in late 2004. A group of 10 U.S. spine surgeons initiated treatment of L5–S1 degenerative disk disease patients to validate the pilot work of Pimenta et al, including ~90 patients in 2005.

The AxiaLIF procedure was released to the spine community in the United States and Europe in 2006 and has accumulated over 6000 procedures to date and generated 17 peer-reviewed original articles and textbook publications. AxiaLIF is one of the most validated and studied MIS lumbar fusion operations: studies include original articles on anatomy, access, biomechanics, functional outcomes, arthrodesis rates, complications for degenerative disk disease, instability, and adult degenerative scoliosis. Although there are no level I studies and most are small series and level II evidence, the amount of data being compiled and reported is impressive.

◆ Preoperative Evaluation

Preoperative planning is extremely important in AxiaLIF, especially with the addition of the two-level procedure. Radiographic images, including a full sacral view, should be used to determine if the anatomy is suitable. The standard field of view for lumbar magnetic resonance imaging (MRI) and computed tomography (CT) must be expanded to include the coccyx to aid in preoperative planning. For the MRI, the patient should be in a prone position with pelvic elevation. Templates have been developed and are now available to help select appropriate patients and to provide implant sizing and trajectory guidance during preoperative planning as well as during surgery. These templates may be used during surgery following a calibration with one of the access instruments not only to help establish the correct sacral entry point and to guide pin trajectory but also, later on in the procedure, to correctly choose the proper implant size for the patient as well as to help determine how deep to drill in the vertebral body based on the chosen implant.

◆ Operative Technique with Anatomical Considerations

Anterior column fusion via AxiaLIF is achieved via a presacral approach first described by Cragg et al.[2] A longitudinal, 2 cm paramedian incision is made ~1 cm off midline. The superior (cephalad) aspect of the incision lies just below the paracoccygeal notch, which is formed by the confluence of the sacrotuberous ligament and sacrospinous ligament.

Careful, blunt finger dissection is employed to progress the incision to the parietal fascia. Once crossed, access is gained to the presacral space. The presacral space is bounded anteriorly by the visceral peritoneum of the mesorectum and posteriorly by the parietal fascia covering the sacrum and coccyx. A filmy complex of areolar tissue and fat lies between these fascial layers. The surgeon must exercise caution during dissection to ensure that neither of the fascial borders is compromised. Breaching the mesorectal visceral fascia can lead to colorectal perforation, whereas crossing the parietal, presacral fascia can expose the underlying venous plexus.

The rectosacral fascia divides the retrorectal space into inferior and superior compartments. It extends from approximately the third or fourth sacral vertebra to the posterior rectal wall, where it terminates 3 to 5 cm above the anorectal junction in the rectal visceral fascia.[5] This fascia can be thick in some patients and require either careful blunt dissection or, in some cases, sharp dissection with an 8 in Kelly/Pean forceps.

Several vascular structures are present in the presacral space, although most are avoided by maintaining a midline approach while traversing the sacrum. The primary exception is the middle sacral artery, which courses from the L5–S1 disc space to the coccyx. Parietal branches of the middle sacral artery proceed to the lateral sacral arteries; visceral branches of the middle sacral artery proceed to the posterior rectum. The path of the middle sacral artery has been shown to be extremely variable, however, and may not be encountered at all during the AxiaLIF procedure.

A detailed examination of presacral anatomy by Yuan et al[6] provides additional insight into proximity of major vascular structures. In this study, the average distance from the sacral midline at the S1–2 level to the left internal iliac artery was 4.3 cm (MRI)/4.0 cm (CT); the average distance to the right internal iliac artery was 3.8 cm (MR/CT). Additionally, the average thickness of the presacral space was found to be 1.2 cm (MR)/1.3 cm (CT). This agrees with Oto et al,whose measurements ranged from 1.06 to 1.62 cm, with significantly thicker presacral widths observed in males (**Fig. 9.1**).[7]

The sympathetic plexus is usually found at the L5–S1 interspace and is not encountered in the typical AxiaLIF surgery, where entry to the sacrum most often occurs at the S1–2 level.

The operative techniques are detailed in prior literature.[8,9] Meticulous preoperative planning must be conducted initially for each patient. Multiplanar imaging facilitated with MRI and plain x-ray films should be utilized for proper patient selection. These studies further delineate the quantity of the mesorectum at plane, the sacral morphology and sagittal trajectory for appropriate guide wire placement. A standard bowel preparation

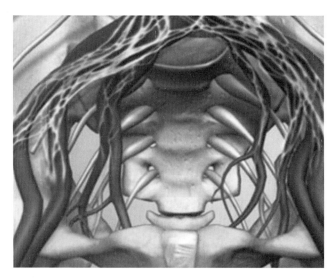

Fig. 9.1   Presacral anatomy—safety zone along midline next to sacrum.

is performed the evening before surgery. In the OR, the patient is to be placed in a prone position on a fluoroscopically compatible surgical table. The sacrum is positioned and raised with flexion and padding of the hips to establish proper posture for axial entry. Optionally, insufflation of air into the rectum is achieved by a rectal catheter, then the operative site is prepared with an adhesive barrier to exclude the perineum.

Minimally invasive axial access to the lower lumbar spine is via the entry site near the apex of the superior gluteal fold. The paracoccygeal ligamentous notch is palpable and is the entry window into the presacral space. A blunt guide pin is advanced to the arch of the caudal sacrum and directed inferiorly under the arch. The guide pin must be carefully advanced and limited upon entry into the pelvis. The guide pin shaft must be deflected downward after traversing the pelvic fascial layer. Biplane fluoroscopy is necessary to ensure safe advancement of the blunt guide wire in the midline presacral space, while the pin position against the sacrum is maintained by downward pressure on the guide pin shaft. When the pin reaches the S1–2 interspace, the trajectory of entry into the anterior lumbar spine is further defined and confirmed by examination of anteroposterior (AP) and lateral fluoroscopy. A sharp beveled guide pin is tapped into the sacrum, followed by sequential dilation to enlarge the soft tissue plane and the entry tract into the sacrum. Axial disk access is accomplished through the 9 mm working channel, and a cannula maintains the trajectory and safe passage of instrumentation into the disk space (**Fig. 9.2**).

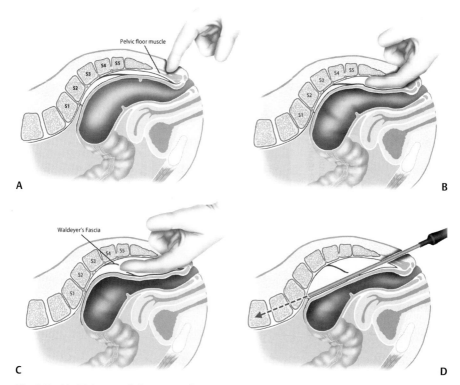

Fig. 9.2 (A–D) Stages of the approach.

A minimally invasive approach for diskectomy follows axial entry. A 3 cm axial diskectomy, end plate preparation, and bone grafting are performed prior to AxiaLIF implantation. Autogenous bone is retrieved during the creation of the intervertebral tract and can be mixed with a bone extender and/or growth factors. It is delivered through an 8 mm bone tamp within a working cannula.

Expandable nitinol curettes are utilized for debulking the nucleus pulposus, the disk tissue is removed, and the end plates abraded within a defined radius to provide a bleeding bed for fusion. The excised disk material is extracted with a series of wire tissue extractors through the same working cannula. A variable pitch and diameter fixation rod is then inserted through an exchange cannula that provides axial distraction and indirect decompression of the L5–S1 segment. An appropriately selected distraction rod is inserted and the transosseous tunnel engaged from the sacrum to the fifth lumbar vertebrae. This differential pitch creates a distraction of the vertebral bodies at a rate dependent on the difference of the thread pitches. Intervertebral fixation is accomplished through the placement of an appropriately sized single fixation rod. After implantation, the access cannula is removed, the skin closed, and an occlusive dressing placed at the percutaneous access site.

If indicated, a mini–open decompression and/or posterior instrumentation with facet screws or pedicle screws, with or without concomitant posterior fusion, can be performed in the routine fashion.

The axial approach to the disk space was a challenge initially for completing a proper diskectomy. A series of retractable nitinol disk cutters evolved that allow the surgeon to place large rigid cutting blades into the disk space through a 9 mm portal to debulk the disk space as well as scrape the cartilage off of the end plates. These cutters initially had single blades and were available in various lengths and angles. The need for a more efficient cutting tool drove the development of the cutter system into four different double-bladed loop-cutter designs varying in length and angle. Each of the four cutters is designed to debulk the nucleus pulposus and lightly abrade the end plates circumferentially up to a 3 cm diameter footprint while creating a bleeding bed for fusion. The radial downcutters are designed to debulk the nucleus pulposus and abrade the caudal end plate, whereas the radial cutters are designed for the cranial end plate. The double-edged blades on each of the cutters allow for cutting in both directions. The next step in the progression of the cutters included the addition of tight disk cutters for collapsed disks where the profile of the standard family of cutters was too large to access the disk space. These tight disk cutters still have two blades but are flat instead of looped, and their stiffness allows them to aggressively abrade the end plates. The profile of these cutters is only 1.3 mm compared with the larger 3 to 4 mm profile of the looped cutters. Tissue extractors (brushes) are used to subsequently grab and remove the material from the disk space that has been cut.

The 3D Axial Rod (TranS1, Wilmington, NC) is the primary implant used for rigid fixation and fusion of the disk space. The thread-on section of the rod that is placed into the L5 vertebral body is a buttress thread with a perpendicular face on the cephalad side of the thread to support compressive forces. The buttress thread on the section of the rod engaged in S1 faces caudally to resist compressive forces in a similar manner. The rod is threaded into the vertebral bodies and has two sections, caudal and cranial. Each section has a different thread pitch and subsequently a

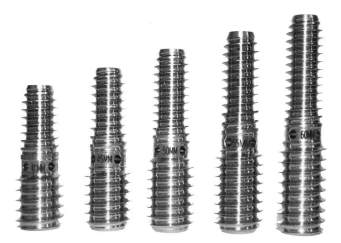

Fig. 9.3 Various 3D Axial Rod sizes (TranS1, Wilmington, NC).

different diameter so that cross threading does not occur. The variable thread pitch creates a distractive force when the rod is threaded into two vertebral bodies simultaneously. This distraction indirectly decompresses the neural foramen and achieves instantaneous fixation of the segment. Early versions of the rod included a small rod and a large rod, with the large rod having larger outer diameters in both sections. The small rod had a cranial diameter of 9 mm and a caudal diameter of 12 mm. The large rod had a cranial diameter of 11 mm and a caudal diameter of 14 mm. The small rod was rarely used early on, and the large rod eventually became the 3D Axial Rod (TranS1). It is offered in various lengths and thread pitch combinations, allowing several options depending on the patient and amount of distraction desired (**Fig. 9.3**).

Initially, the approach was used to treat only the L5–S1 disk space, but it has advanced to allow access, preparation, and implantation of the L4–5 disk space through the same incision. Due to the unique surgical approach and the addition of the two-level system, preoperative planning, access technique, diskectomy, and fixation methods have all undergone some transformation as the procedure has matured and evolved over the past few years.

The AxiaLIF 2L Rod (TranS1) (**Fig. 9.4**) consists of two titanium implants that seat together creating a rigid fixation from L4 to S1. The first rod is placed at L4–5 and distracts the disk space using the differential thread pitch similar to the 3D Axial Rod. The second rod (the S1 Rod) has one threaded section and a tapered shaft at the tip that engages the L4–5 Rod. Distraction at L5–S1 is created by the S1 Rod turning against the L4–5 Rod, thus separating the L5 body from the S1 body and increasing the disk height. Initially, the L4–5 Rod had the same diameters as the small 3D Axial Rod. These diameters (L4 = 9 mm and L5 = 12 mm) were insufficient for proper fixation across the L4–5 space. Therefore the diameters of the system were increased to the current dimensions. The L4 portion of the rod now has a diameter of 11 mm. The L5 portion of the rod has a diameter of 13 mm, and the S1 Rod has a diameter of 15.5 mm. The L4–5 rods are offered in various lengths and thread pitch combinations,

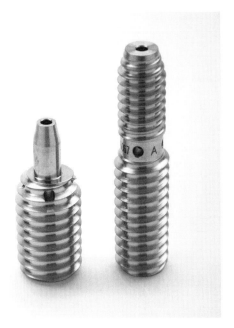

Fig. 9.4 The AxiaLIF-2L Rod assembly. The S1 Rod is on the left and the L4-5 Rod is on the right. (TranS1, Wilmington, NC).

whereas the S1 Rod is offered only in several lengths due to the manner in which it distracts.

◆ Discussion

Patient Outcomes

Due to the minimally invasive nature of the procedure, AxiaLIF stabilization has potential benefits when compared with other surgical options. The rate of fusion observed for single AxiaLIF L5–S1 fusion procedures ranged from 82 to 91% at 1 and 2 years postoperatively[3,10–13] (**Fig. 9.5**). These results are comparable at 2 years to an open ALIF performed with and without bone morphogenetic protein, with reported fusion rates ranging from 68 to 88%.[3,11,12] Other multiple ALIF clinical studies have demonstrated similar fusion rates, ranging from 68 to 96%.[14,15] Comparatively, the fusion rate for the AxiaLIF System was well aligned with conventional interbody fusion techniques, and performed superior to allograft bone dowels, while also proving equivalent to fusions enhanced with bone morphogenetic proteins.[11,14,15] The results reported for transforaminal lumbar interbody fusion (TLIF) with bone morphogenetic protein have demonstrated a fusion success rate of 92%.[16] However, for interbody fusion procedures that require removal of surrounding ligamentous structures or the facet joint, implant migration and a reduction in biomechanical stability are potential risks.

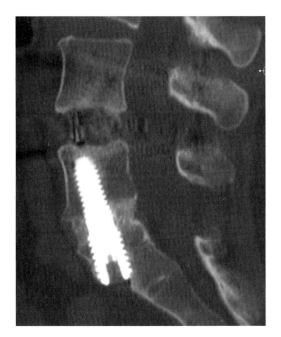

Fig. 9.5   Solid arthrodesis through disk space. Notice cage above does not show bridging bone.

The advantage of the AxiaLIF System (TranS1) is that posterior implant migration is not possible because it does not disrupt the facet joint, nor does it remove surrounding ligamentous tissue that would allow space for expulsion or migration to occur. Furthermore, it traverses the intervertebral disk space, resisting sheer forces, and is anchored in the superior and inferior vertebral bodies surrounding the disk, creating greater resistance to migration and expulsion. Compromise of the annular tissue for surgical implantation of conventional interbody fusion procedures can potentially destabilize the spinal segment. Maintenance of these structures provides improved stability and immobility to the spinal segment to allow for bone incorporation during the fusion process, with a reduced risk of excessive motion and instability during healing.[17]

Through the naturally existing presacral fat pad, ready access can be gained to the disk space while completely avoiding the anterior abdominopelvic cavity, great vessels, nerves, muscles, and facet joints. For larger, overweight patients, access to the lumbar spine via the presacral axial approach is ideal because it allows for less tissue infiltration than that of an anterior approach, resulting in fewer complications, less tissue destruction, and less risk of infection, and it will not require specialized insertion tools. Additionally, in obese patients an axial surgical approach to the spine provides a margin of safety superior to that of traditional anterior lumbar interbody fusion (ALIF), posterior lumbar interbody fusion (PLIF), and TLIF approaches due to the larger presacral fat pad surrounding the rectal region and protecting the neural structures and rectum.

Numerous prospective and retrospective clinical studies have demonstrated the AxiaLIF minimally invasive interbody fusion to be a viable alternative for providing anterior column support for long-segment fusions to the sacrum.[11,18,19] The procedure has demonstrated equivalent fusion rates for the L5–S1 disk space while being associated with less risk of neural damage and loss of stability due to its tissue-sparing capabilities. Multiple-level fusions (L4–S1) have since been incorporated into the AxiaLIF System and have demonstrated positive fusion outcomes. Preliminary studies have demonstrated 90% fusion rates at 12 months postoperatively with significant reductions in pain, with 17.6% reductions in the Oswestry Disability Index (ODI) scores.[18] However, radiolucencies were identified radiographically at the distal tip of the L4 AxiaLIF rod as well as the screw tips of the posterior supplemental fixation, with no evidence of subsidence in a few of these patients. Additionally noted for the patients exhibiting radiolucencies were clear demarcated margins of new bone growth surrounding the vicinity of radiolucencies at the 12-month time period.

With respect to the radiolucencies observed with the two-level AxiaLIF fusion procedure, there is a cascade of biomechanical events related to fusion healing that may explain the existence of some radiolucencies in the presence of very successful fusion outcomes. Bone is a responsive viscoelastic tissue that forms in response to increased stresses. It resorbs in response to decreased stresses and/or micromotion and has approximately a 12- to 24-week turnover rate.[20] The process of bone healing occurs in three distinct but overlapping phases: (1) the inflammatory phase, (2) the repair phase, and (3) the late remodeling stage. This entire healing process occurs within the first 12 to 24 weeks postoperatively.[21] However, factors related to lifestyle (i.e., smoking, body mass, diabetes, medications, etc.) can alter and delay the healing timeline.

Ideally, supplemental fixation should be placed at every level of a fusion to provide uniformly distributed stabilization across each fusion site. This would distribute the stresses uniformly and over a greater surface area throughout the anterior and posterior fixation (rod and pedicle screws), thus reducing the stresses at the bone and implant interface at each level. By skipping a level of fixation, additional stress is transferred to the superior portion of the implant and bony interface, increasing the risk of additional micromotion, and stresses are placed upon the bone at that region of stress transfer. Additionally, the lack of multisegmental points of pedicle screw fixation across each fusion site poses a challenging biomechanical environment. The end result is a longer lever arm across the L4–S1 spinal segment, contributing to added stress and micromotion transfer to the upper-level point of fixation (L4 vertebra). It is very likely that the added stress and micromotion at the upper pedicle screws further contribute to the radiolucent cascade during the early stages of fusion healing.

Complications

As of November 30, 2008, a total of 5290 AxiaLIF surgeries had been completed. The total known complication rate at this time was 1.08%, whereas the serious complication rate was 0.79% (data provided by TranS1). The most prevalent complication is bowel injury (0.59%). There have been no reports of deaths or permanent injury. This compares favorably to other approaches to interbody spinal fusion.

PLIF provides for diskectomy, interbody placement, and rigid fixation through one incision. Direct decompression can also be achieved, but there are several complications associated with this technique. Okuda et al[22] noted dural tears (7.6%), pedicle screw malposition (2.8%), increased leg pain (0.8%), slight/severe motor loss (2.4%/3.6%), and permanent motor loss (1.6%) as reported complications. Park et al[23] reported a 9.1% complication rate for PLIF in a comparison between PLIF and TLIF. Prior posterior surgery increases the difficulty of this approach significantly.

ALIF provides the most generous access to the L5–S1 disk space and allows for optimally sized interbody insertion. It does not require dissection of spinal muscles and is associated with little blood loss. Its use is best limited to cases without prior abdominal surgery; revisions can be especially challenging, with vascular complication rates exceeding 50%.[24] Hynes et al[25] observed a 10% rate of vascular injuries and a 1.1% rate of retrograde ejaculation in index ALIF surgeries. Infection and injuries to the genitofemoral nerve have also been reported in the literature.

TLIF allows for direct decompression (at least on one side) and requires minimal retraction of the neural elements to gain access to the disk space. The PLL is preserved, as well as other support structures in the midline. The L5–S1 disk space can be challenging in TLIF, however, particularly in cases of spondylolisthesis. Eckman et al[26] reported a significant rate of injury to nerve roots (27%). Other complications include radiculopathy (4%),[27] low fusion rate,[28] and poorly prepared end plate.[29] Khan et al[32] reviewed incidence of dural tears in 3183 cases. An incidence of 7.6% was observed in primary lumbar surgeries; this number increased to 15.9% in revision surgery.

In spite of its growing popularity, little has been reported in the medical literature about lateral approaches to lumbar interbody fusion. The lateral (transpsoas) approach avoids the spinal muscle dissection required for posterior approaches and reduces the risk of vascular injury associated with the anterior approach. The lateral approach is not feasible at L5–S1 because the iliac crest blocks access to the disk space. This is also true for the L4–5 level in a meaningful percentage of patients. Prolonged retraction of the genitofemoral nerve (both from lateral positioning as well as from retraction) can be problematic, and patients must be repositioned for insertion of posterior fixation. Bergey et al[30] noted postoperative paresthesias in the groin and thigh region (30%). Bertagnoli and Vazquez[31] described neurapraxia in the psoas as well (80%). Furthermore, anatomically there is significantly greater risk of nerve damage via a direct lateral approach at L4–5 than at the other more cranial levels.

Revision Techniques

In cases that require postoperative intervention, the implant can either be revised or removed. In cases of pseudarthrosis, a posterolateral fusion can be conducted, or interbody cages filled with bone graft to facilitate fusion can be placed around the fusion rod (8 mm diameter in the disk space) through either an index ALIF or PLIF procedure. In cases where removal of the fusion implant is required, it can be simply removed via the implantation tract utilizing the same access path and instrumentation that were used initially (**Fig. 9.6**).

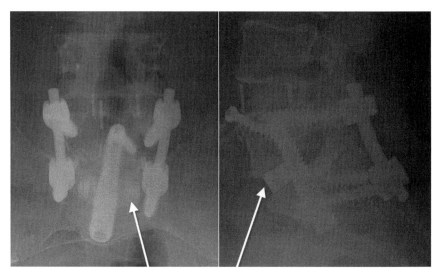

Fig. 9.6 Transforaminal lumbar interbody fusion cage (shown by white arrows) in front of the AxiaLIF rod for pseudarthrosis revision.

Avoidance, Detection, and Treatment of Colorectal Injuries in AxiaLIF Surgery

The most significant complication associated with AxiaLIF surgery is rectal perforation. Although the rate of this injury is low (0.59%), the severity of the injury is disproportionately high. This is due to its being historically addressed via temporary diverting colostomy/ileostomy, an outcome that has both lifestyle and psychosocial implications for the patient.

As experience has been gained with the surgery, several technique modifications have been made to mitigate this complication:

- Full MRI to the tip of the coccyx
  - Evaluate size and extent of presacral space
  - Check for aberrant vasculature
  - Confirm trajectory
- Full bowel prep
  - Ensures rectum is mobile
  - Decreases chance of contamination in case of injury
  - Includes Foley in rectum
  - Includes air injected into rectum (under live fluoroscopy to prevent distention of rectum), which allows identification of landmarks and presacral space
- Blunt finger dissection
  - Mobilizes rectum from sacrum
  - Allows tactile feel for confirmation of proper dissection plane

Instrument changes have also been implemented:

- Fixation wire
  - Secures the exchange cannula to the sacrum and ensures the exchange cannula's close apposition to the sacrum to reduce tissue migration into the operative corridor
- Blunt exchange cannula
  - Reduces likelihood of tissue being "pinched" between the sacrum and cannula

A review of all AxiaLIF rectal perforations with consulting colorectal surgeons suggests early detection may be the key to reducing the percentage of perforations treated via stoma. An injury detected at the time of surgery in a patient with recent bowel prep can be treated much like the injuries observed in colonoscopy: nothing by mouth, antibiotic regimen, and primary repair of the defect if required.

This is especially true for AxiaLIF surgery, where the injury is more likely to occur in the extraperitoneal portion of the rectum. Intraabdominal injuries are less likely to benefit from this treatment regimen but are also less likely to be experienced in AxiaLIF surgery given the location of the peritoneal reflection in most patients at or above the point at which the AxiaLIF system docks to the sacrum.

Rectal defects as a result of AxiaLIF surgery can be quickly and easily identified with either rigid or flexible sigmoidoscopy. Many AxiaLIF surgeons have begun to incorporate this type of postop examination into their surgical routine.

TranS1 has begun to recommend that spine surgeons consult with local general/colorectal surgeons prior to the first AxiaLIF surgery. The spine surgeon can receive advice on bowel prep and antibiotics, while the general/colorectal surgeon can become acquainted with the type and location of injuries that might occur during the surgery. Finally, the two can agree on a treatment protocol and postop call to action according to patient warning signs. Going forward, these steps may greatly reduce the already low rate of colorectal complications during AxiaLIF surgery.

Future Developments

A modular rod system is in development that takes advantage of all the benefits of the approach and expands on the potential of the 3D Axial Rod. The new system will allow for more precise distraction of each disk space and bone grafting of the disk space following distraction, and it will offer the same the rigid fixation achieved with the current system.

Although the minimally invasive axial access to the L5–S1 and L4–5 disk space is beneficial for lumbosacral fusion as described previously, it is ideally suited for a nucleus replacement device. The preservation of the integrity of the annulus translates to minimal risk of implant expulsion, lower morbidity with respect to the approach, and no destabilization of the spinal unit due to the nondisruption of surrounding tissue. The TranS1 Percutaneous Nucleus Replacement (PNR) implant takes advantage of these benefits as it is inserted in a similar manner as the 3D Axial Rod. The PNR is a motion-preserving device that is designed to restore disk height and allow normal loading patterns through proper tensioning of the disk. Two anchors are threaded into each vertebral body on either side of the disk space. The nucleus

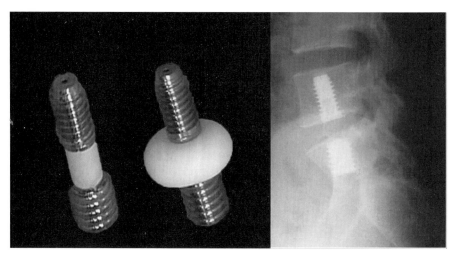

Fig. 9.7   Prosthetic Nuclear Replacement (PNR, TranS1, Wilmington, NC).

implant inserter is then placed through one anchor and into the more distal anchor. A distraction handle and shaft mechanism distract the disk space utilizing the vertebral body anchors prior to insertion of the nucleus filler material. The in situ curing silicone rubber is infused through the delivery device and expands the silicone rubber membrane and protective polyester jacket within the denucleated disk space until it is filled. The mixed materials cross-link to form a radiopaque, low-durometer rubber with high mechanical properties and excellent resistance to permanent deformation. The silicone material acts as an incompressible fluid within the annulus, transferring compressive loads on the disk to hoop stress on the annulus similar to the way in which healthy nucleus acts during loading (**Fig. 9.7**).

The TranS1 Partial Disc Replacement (PDR) is a motion-preserving or supported nucleus system that is metal on metal with an in situ formed bumper around the central support. It is delivered through the same presacral access as the 3D Axial Rod, and the design of the device allows it to function when the annulus has been compromised or is degenerated to a point that it no longer properly functions. The PDR is designed to eliminate pain by reestablishing the normal disk height while allowing motion similar to a total disk replacement. Unlike traditional TDR devices, the approach used to implant the PDR maintains all the ligaments and surrounding soft tissue structures for better stability.

◆ Conclusions

The novel yet simple axial approach to the lower lumbar spine has demonstrated reliable and reproducible safety and efficacy when compared with established ALIF, PLIF, and TLIF approaches. Advances in technology have improved the safety of surgical interventions, limiting morbidity associated with larger procedures by applying the concepts of minimally invasive surgery. With recently developed minimally invasive spinal surgical techniques, these procedures involve less postoperative pain, shorter hospital stay, and fewer medications than with conventional surgery. The axial approach toward spinal fusion requires significantly less tissue destruction and can be placed via a minimally invasive approach to the spine, leaving the surrounding supportive bone intact. With the development of axial nuclear replacement and axial mechanical disk replacement, this may prove to be a utilitarian approach to treat multiple pathologies in different stages of the degenerative cascade of the lower lumbar spine in the future.

References

1. Smith MD, Bohlman HH. Spondylolisthesis treated by a single-stage operation combining decompression with in situ posterolateral and anterior fusion: an analysis of eleven patients who had long-term follow-up. J Bone Joint Surg Am 1990;72:415–421

2. Cragg A, Carl A, Casteneda F, Dickman C, Guterman L, Oliveira C. New percutaneous access method for minimally invasive anterior lumbosacral surgery. J Spinal Disord Tech 2004;17:21–28

3. Pimenta L, Guerrero L, Cragg A, Diaz R. Minimal invasive percutaneous presacral axial lumbar fusion (AxiaLIF): prospective clinical and radiographic results after 30 months follow-up. Section on Disorders of the Spine and Peripheral Nerves, Congress of Neurosurgeons, Chicago, IL, October 7–12, 2006

4. Levy, E. New minimally invasive surgical technique moves lumbar spinal fusion to the cath lab. Cath Lab Digest 2005;(August) Special Clinical Issue

5. Carl A, Ledet E, Oliveira C, et al. Colorectal disease: percutaneous axial lumbar spine surgery. In: Perez-Cruet MJ, Khoo LT, Fessler RG, eds. An Anatomic Approach to Minimally Invasive Spine Surgery. St. Louis, MO: Quality Medical Publishing; 2006:654–670

6. Yuan PS, Day TF, Albert TJ, et al. Anatomy of the percutaneous presacral space for a novel fusion technique. J Spinal Disord Tech 2006;19:237–241

7. Oto A, Peynircioglu B, Eryilmaz M, Besim A, Sürücü HS, Celik HH. Determination of the width of the presacral space on magnetic resonance imaging. Clin Anat 2004;17:14–16

8. Cragg A, Carl A, Ledet E, Diaz R, Pimenta L. Percutaneous Axial Lumbar Spine Surgery: An Anatomical Approach to Minimally Invasive Spine Surgery. St. Louis, MO: Quality Medical; 2006:653–670

9. Marotta N, Cosar M, Pimenta L, Khoo LT. A novel minimally invasive presacral approach and instrumentation technique for anterior L5–S1 intervertebral discectomy and fusion: technical description and case presentations. Neurosurg Focus 2006;20:E9

10. Pimenta L, Bellera F, Carl A, Ledet E, Cragg A. New percutaneous access method and implant for L4–S1 spinal fusion surgery. Presented at AANS, Session 118 New and Evolving MIS Techniques: Drs. Fessler, Pimenta, Smith, and Isaacs; Orlando, FL; May 1–6, 2004

11. Aryan HE, Newman CB, Gold JJ, Acosta FL Jr, Coover C, Ames CP. Percutaneous axial lumbar interbody fusion (AxiaLIF) of the L5–S1 segment: initial clinical and radiographic experience. Minim Invasive Neurosurg 2008;51:225–230

12. Bradley W, Roush T, Hisey M, Ohnmeiss D. Minimally invasive trans-sacral approach to L5–S1 interbody fusion: technique and clinical results. SAS Global Symposium on Motion Preservation Technology; 8th Annual Meeting; Miami, FL; May 6–9, 2008

13. Tobler W, Bohinski R. Experience in 150 cases with the TranS1 minimally invasive fusion technique at L5–S1. Global Symposium on Motion Preservation Technology; 8th Annual Meeting; Miami, FL; May 6–9, 2008

14. Burkus JK. Bone morphogenetic proteins in anterior lumbar interbody fusion: old techniques and new technologies. Invited submission from the Joint Section Meeting on Disorders of the Spine and Peripheral Nerves, March 2004. J Neurosurg Spine 2004;1:254–260

15. Burkus JK, Dorchak JD, Sanders DL. Radiographic assessment of interbody fusion using recombinant human bone morphogenetic protein type 2. Spine (Phila Pa 1976) 2003;28:372–377

16. Salehi SA, Tawk R, Ganju A, LaMarca F, Liu JC, Ondra SL. Transforaminal lumbar interbody fusion: surgical technique and results in 24 patients. Neurosurgery 2004;54:368–374

17. Akesen B, Wu C, Mehbod AA, Transfeldt EE. Biomechanical evaluation of paracoccygeal transsacral fixation. J Spinal Disord Tech 2008;21:39–44

18. Pimenta L, Pesantez A, Lhamby J, Oliveira L, Schaffa T, Coutinho E. Two levels presacral Axial Lumbar Interbody Fusion (AxiaLIF): a prospective 12 months follow up: clinical and radiological results. Global Symposium on Motion Preservation Technology; 8th Annual Meeting; Miami, FL; May 6–9, 2008

19. Anand N, Baron EM, Thaiyananthan G, Khalsa K, Goldstein TB. Minimally invasive multilevel percutaneous correction and fusion for adult lumbar degenerative scoliosis: a technique and feasibility study. J Spinal Disord Tech 2008;21:459–467

20. Wolff J. Des Gesetz der Transformation der Knochen. Berlin: A. Hirschwald, 1892. Translated by P. Manquet and R. Furlong as The Law of Bone Remodelling. Berlin: Springer, 1986.

21. Kalfas IH. Principles of bone healing. Neurosurg Focus 2001;10:E1

22. Okuda S, Miyauchi A, Oda T, Haku T, Yamamoto T, Iwasaki M. Surgical complications of posterior lumbar interbody fusion with total facetectomy in 251 patients. J Neurosurg Spine 2006;4:304–309

23. Park JS, Kim YB, Hong HJ, Hwang SN. Comparison between posterior and transforaminal approaches for lumbar interbody fusion. J Korean Neurosurg Soc 2005;37:340–344

24. Nguyen HV, Akbarnia BA, van Dam BE, et al. Anterior exposure of the spine for removal of lumbar interbody devices and implants. Spine (Phila Pa 1976) 2006;31:2449–2453

25. Hynes R, Wasselle J, Velez D. Complications of the lumbar anterior surgical approach for artificial disc replacement of the lumbar spine. Spine J 2005;5:S64–S65

26. Eckman W, McMillen M, Hester L. Incidence and etiology of transient nerve root injury with lumbar transforaminal surgery. Spine J 2007;7:126S–127S

27. Schwender JD, Holly LT, Rouben DP, Foley KT. Minimally invasive transforaminal lumbar interbody fusion (TLIF): technical feasibility and initial results. J Spinal Disord Tech 2005;18(Suppl):S1–S6

28. Poh S, Yue WM, Chen LT, et al. Clinical and radiological evaluation of transforaminal lumbar interbody fusion at 2 years follow-up. Spine J 2007;7:25S

29. Javernick MA, Kuklo TR, Polly DW Jr. Transforaminal lumbar interbody fusion: unilateral versus bilateral disk removal—an in vivo study. Am J Orthop 2003;32:344–348

30. Bergey DL, Villavicencio AT, Goldstein T, Regan JJ. Endoscopic lateral transpsoas approach to the lumbar spine. Spine (Phila Pa 1976) 2004;29:1681–1688

31. Bertagnoli R, Vazquez RJ. The Anterolateral TransPsoatic Approach (ALPA): a new technique for implanting prosthetic disc-nucleus devices. J Spinal Disord Tech 2003;16:398–404

32. Khan MH, Rihn J, Steele G, et al. Postoperative management protocol for incidental dural tears during degenerative lumbar spine surgery: a review of 3,183 consecutive degenerative lumbar cases. Spine (Phila Pa 1976) 2006;31:2609–2613

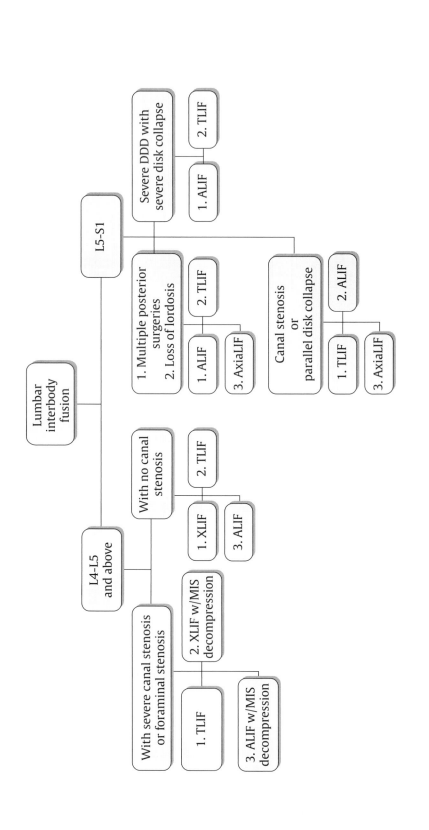

10

Minimally Invasive Lumbar Interbody Fusion: Choosing Between Approaches

Amjad N. Anaizi, Jean-Marc Voyadzis, and Faheem A. Sandhu

In 2001 the Swedish Lumbar Spine Study Group confirmed that lumbar spine arthrodesis was superior to conservative management of debilitating low back pain.[1] In addition to alleviating mechanical low back pain and radicular pain, restoration of normal lumbar lordosis and overall sagittal balance is crucial in ensuring lasting pain relief and improved quality of life. To this end, interbody fusion techniques have been used with increasing frequency and offer several advantages over traditional posterior spinal fusion techniques. The increased surface area for fusion and ability to place the graft material under compressive forces should help facilitate fusion. In addition, the ability to reestablish normal disk space height allows for indirect decompression of foraminal stenosis.

The concept of spinal fusion was first introduced in the early 1900s by Albee and Hibbs.[2,3] They described posterior spinal fusion for management of spinal deformity associated with Pott disease. The first description of an interbody fusion was by Capener and colleagues in the 1930s.[4] This was an anterior lumbar interbody fusion (ALIF) via a transabdominal approach for treatment of spondylolisthesis. Years later, in 1953, Cloward described the posterior lumbar interbody fusion (PLIF), allowing for an interbody fusion through a true midline posterior approach.[5] Harms and colleagues later introduced the transforaminal lumbar interbody fusion, with the goal of accomplishing an interbody fusion as in the PLIF but through a unilateral posterolateral approach, obviating the need for significant retraction of the neural elements and hence decreasing the potential for neural injury.[6] The eXtreme Lateral Interbody Fusion (XLIF, NuVasive, Inc., San Diego, CA), described by Pimenta in 2001, is a true lateral approach through the retroperitoneal space to the spine.[7] XLIF offers many of the same advantages of ALIF while decreasing some of the inherent risks of an anterior approach to the spine. Pimenta also introduced the axial lumbar interbody fusion (AxiaLIF, TranS1, Wilmington, NC), an approach that utilizes the presacral space as an access corridor to the L5–S1 interspace.[8] This evolution in spinal fusion has been driven by a desire to minimize morbidity and collateral damage to the surrounding anatomical structures of the spine.

The indications for lumbar interbody fusion have expanded since they were first described for the management of spondylolisthesis. Patients with recurrent lumbar disk herniations, postlaminectomy syndrome, and those with axial back pain secondary to degenerative disk disease are now routinely managed with interbody fusion. Patients at high risk for pseudarthrosis or those undergoing reoperations for pseudarthrosis are often also best managed with interbody fusion.[9]

This chapter reviews the minimally invasive interbody fusion techniques, highlights their advantages, and discusses their indications. The chapter is summarized in the form of a decision-making algorithm designed to help surgeons select the appropriate minimally invasive interbody fusion technique for various clinical scenarios.

◆ Operative Techniques

Minimally Invasive Transforaminal Lumbar Interbody Fusion with Percutaneous Pedicle Screw Stabilization

The transforaminal lumbar interbody fusion (TLIF) is a common procedure performed for the management of a variety of pathologies requiring lumbar arthrodesis. Through a unilateral approach (preferably the side with radicular symptoms) a hemilaminectomy and facetectomy are performed, providing access to the interbody space. A complete diskectomy and end plate preparation are performed, followed by insertion of an interbody graft, which achieves anterior column support. Pedicle screws are inserted and the construct is compressed to facilitate fusion across the interbody graft and reestablish lumbar lordosis.

The minimally invasive variation on the TLIF procedure (MI-TLIF) was first described in 2003 by Foley et al and has since become an increasingly popular method of lumbar arthrodesis, offering the advantages of an open TLIF through a smaller exposure.[10,11] As opposed to the open approach, the MI-TLIF is performed through a unilateral paramedian incision. Tubular dilators are utilized to minimize injury to the paraspinal musculature. Contralateral percutaneous pedicle screws may be inserted to achieve distraction. Bony decompression, diskectomy, end plate preparation, and interbody graft insertion are achieved through a muscle splitting approach. Ipsilateral pedicle screws are inserted and the construct compressed as in the open approach.[10]

The minimally invasive TLIF has several important advantages over the open technique. A paramedian approach with removal of the pars interarticularis and total facetectomy allow for a complete decompression of the ipsilateral neural structures and avoid undue retraction of the thecal sac during placement of the bone graft. Furthermore, the structural integrity of the midline osteoligamentous structures is maintained, and the placement of contralateral percutaneous instrumentation minimizes tissue disruption, particularly the facet capsules. The side of the approach should always be ipsilateral to the patient's radicular symptoms. In cases of severe canal stenosis, decompressive laminectomy can be performed, the spinous process undercut, and the contralateral lamina drilled to achieve bilateral decompression of the spinal canal. In cases of severe bilateral foraminal stenosis, a minimally invasive decompression can be performed through a separate contralateral incision using tubular retractors through which pedicle screws can also be placed. Revision surgery is not made more complicated by a minimally invasive approach. In fact, a paramedian/MI approach for revision surgery is advantageous because it avoids traversing scar tissue, which is unavoidable with exposure through a traditional midline incision.

There are certain disadvantages to the TLIF and its MI counterpart. One important limitation is the difficulty involved in placing a large interbody graft when needed to reestablish normal disk space height and lordosis. It is also difficult to ensure that the graft rests anterior to the instantaneous axis of rotation. Sufficient anterior placement of the graft is crucial in reestablishing normal lumbar lordosis following compression of the dorsal fusion construct. A contraindication to this procedure is the presence of a conjoined nerve root within the foramen.[11] Although this is an exceedingly rare occurrence, it is one for which there should be a thorough evaluation on preoperative imaging. Attempts to retract the neural elements of conjoined roots for graft placement carry a significant risk of neurological injury.[11] If this is appreciated preoperatively, a contralateral TLIF or alternative approach should be considered.

Although the MI-TLIF with percutaneous pedicle screws is a relatively new approach, there is early evidence supporting its effectiveness. Lowe et al published a series of 40 patients who underwent minimally invasive TLIF and were followed for an average of 36 months.[12] Patients in this series had a confirmed fusion rate of 90%, a significant reduction in pain, and improvement in the Oswestry Disability Index. Schwender et al evaluated the effectiveness of this technique in a series of 49 patients with a minimum of 18 months follow-up.[13] In this series, all patients had solid fusion based on radiographic criteria at last follow-up. Patients also had significant improvements in average visual analog pain scale and Oswestry Disability Index. Jang and Lee had similar results in their series of 23 patients who underwent an MI-TLIF with ipsilateral pedicle screw and contralateral facet screw stabilization.[14]

The indications for a minimally invasive TLIF mirror those for an open TLIF and include degenerative disk disease, grade 1–2 spondylolisthesis associated with mechanical back pain or radicular pain, and recurrent disk herniations with or without mechanical back pain. It is a particularly ideal technique in patients with back pain with unilateral radiculopathy from severe foraminal stenosis or recurrent disk herniations with significant lumbar stenosis (**Fig. 10.1**).

Minimally Invasive Lateral Interbody Fusion with Percutaneous Pedicle Screw Stabilization

The eXtreme Lateral Interbody Fusion (XLIF) technique was first described by Pimenta in 2001 as a modification of the traditional retroperitoneal approach to the lumbar spine.[15] This approach shares many of the advantages of the traditional retroperitoneal exposure in that it provides direct visualization of the disk space and vertebral body, allows for the insertion of a large interbody spacer, and can provide indirect decompression of central and foraminal stenosis. Further, it eliminates many of the disadvantages of an open anterior approach, including the potential need for an access surgeon, risk of

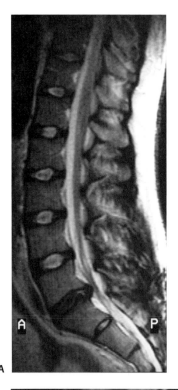

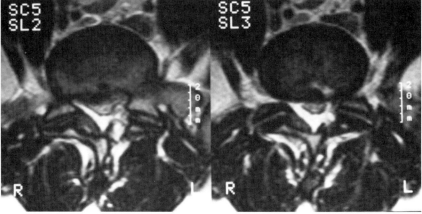

Fig. 10.1 A 36-year-old man presented with long-standing back pain and left leg pain with a history of previous L5–S1 diskectomy. **(A)** Preoperative sagittal and **(B)** axial magnetic resonance images showed degenerative disk disease at the L5–S1 level with left foraminal stenosis. The patient failed to improve with conservative management and underwent a left-sided L5–S1 minimally invasive transforaminal lumbar interbody fusion with percutaneous screw stabilization.

vascular or sympathetic nerve injury, and anterior longitudinal ligament disruption. As a result of the transpsoas tubular dilation, there is a risk of injury to the nerve roots of the lumbosacral plexus, particularly at L4–5. However, this is mitigated through the use of real-time intraoperative neural monitoring systems. The XLIF technique is limited to interspaces above the iliac crest and is not applicable to L5–S1 or L4–5 in some cases.

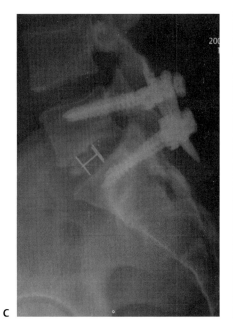
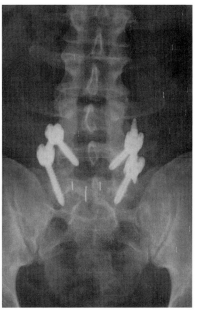

C

D

Fig. 10.1 (*continued*)   Postoperative AP (**C**) and lateral x-rays (**D**) demonstrating placement of the interbody spacer and instrumentation. The patient had significant relief of his back and left leg pain following surgery.

The patient is placed in the lateral decubitus position and secured to the operating table with tape. To enter the retroperitoneal space we utilize a single incision technique centered over the disk space of interest using lateral fluoroscopy. For multilevel cases, the incision is placed in the midpoint of the operative area. The external, internal oblique, and transversus abdominis are split along their normal course to gain entry into the retroperitoneal space. The psoas muscle is directly visualized, and blunt dissection can be performed to facilitate positioning of the initial dilator. Continuous electromyographic (EMG) monitoring, while the dilator is passed through the psoas muscle and docked onto the disk space of interest, is used to avoid injury to the lumbar nerve roots. Sequential dilators are then passed through the psoas muscle, and finally a retractor is secured in place. An annulotomy, complete diskectomy, and careful end plate preparation are subsequently performed followed by insertion of an interbody graft.

The lateral interbody fusion technique accomplishes lumbar arthrodesis with the minimum possible disruption of normal spinal anatomy. This approach minimizes perturbation of the posterior osseous and ligamentous structures in addition to the posterior musculature. It also maintains the integrity of both the anterior and posterior longitudinal ligaments. A true lateral approach allows for placement of a large interbody graft, thus maximizing fusion potential while also achieving indirect decompression of the neural foramen by restoring disk height. The lateral interbody fusion offers many of the advantages of an ALIF while minimizing the attendant risks to the peritoneum, the great vessels, and the sympathetic plexus.

The lateral interbody fusion approach does have its limitations. L5–S1 cannot be reached due to the presence of the iliac crest. Starting in a lateral position often requires that patients be repositioned for supplemental posterior stabilization. Additionally, there is a risk of injury to the lumbosacral plexus and genitofemoral nerve during the transpsoas dissection, particularly at L4–5. This can cause weakness and painful leg dysesthesias, respectively. The peritoneal cavity can also be violated, leading to bowel injury.

The indications for lateral interbody fusion include degenerative disk disease, grade 1–2 spondylolisthesis, and recurrent lumbar disk herniations without significant canal stenosis. Patients with degenerative disk disease and unilateral disk space collapse with moderate foraminal stenosis and radiculopathy are ideal candidates for this technique. In a patient with concurrent canal stenosis, a minimally invasive TLIF may prove to be a more appropriate technique, given that it provides the ability for bilateral decompressive laminectomy without additional exposure. However, the lateral interbody fusion can be supplemented with a minimally invasive decompressive laminectomy at the same setting that posterior stabilization is performed, without the need for additional incisions. The lateral trajectory of the lateral interbody fusion technique may also prove to be ideal for patients with a history of prior posterior spinal surgery because it avoids related scar tissue (**Fig. 10.2**).

Anterior Lumbar Interbody Fusion with Percutaneous Pedicle Screw Stabilization

Since its introduction in the 1930s for the management of spondylolisthesis, ALIF has become a commonly used technique to achieve lumbar arthrodesis. ALIF is a direct anterior approach to the lumbar spine that avoids disruption of posterior spinal anatomy. Over the years several variations on the traditional ALIF have been developed, including the mini–open ALIF, the laparoscopic ALIF, and the endoscopic retroperitoneal ALIF. We consider all these approaches, including the traditional open ALIF, to be minimally invasive because they minimize disruption of the normal spinal anatomy. A discussion on the variations of the ALIF technique is beyond the scope of this chapter. This is an approach with very important and unique advantages and disadvantages that must be thoroughly considered by the spine surgeons.

After induction of general endotracheal anesthesia the patient is placed in the supine position. The abdomen is widely prepped and draped in a sterile fashion. A paramedian incision is made and retroperitoneal dissection performed. The anterior spinal anatomy is defined and the disk space exposed. This may require retraction and mobilization of the great vessels, especially at the L4–5 disk space. A complete diskectomy is performed, with care taken to avoid damage to the end plate. Once sufficient end plate preparation has been performed, a suitable interbody graft is inserted. Appropriate placement of the graft is confirmed with fluoroscopy. The incision is irrigated and closed in the standard fashion. The patient is then placed in the prone position and percutaneous pedicle screw fixation is performed. This may also be performed in a second stage.

We consider ALIF to be a minimally invasive procedure because of its near complete preservation of normal spinal anatomy, only requiring disruption of the anterior longitudinal ligament, annulus, and disk for insertion of the intervertebral graft. Disk space

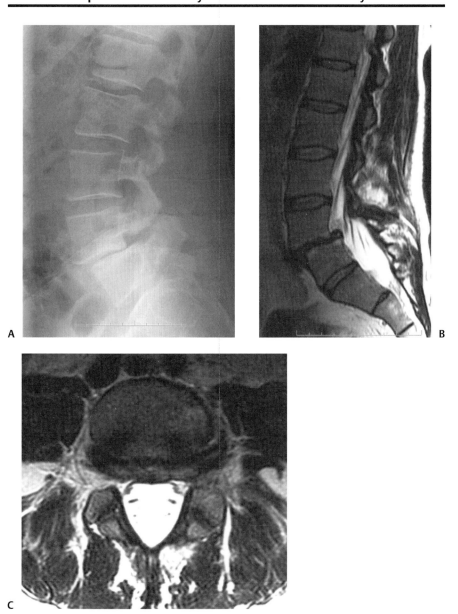

Fig. 10.2 A 47-year-old man presented with long-standing low back pain that progressed to bilateral lower extremity pain that was worse on the left. **(A)** Lateral lumbar x-ray revealed grade 2 spondylolisthesis at L4–5 that did not reduce on flexion/extension imaging (not shown). **(B,C)** Magnetic resonance imaging of the lumbar spine showed grade 2 spondylolisthesis at L4–5 and bilateral foraminal stenosis, worse on the left. After failure of conservative management, he underwent an L4–5 lateral interbody fusion followed by percutaneous screw stabilization. (*continued*)

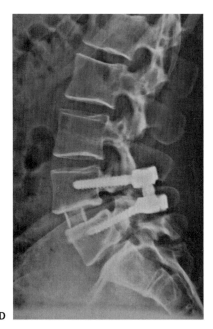
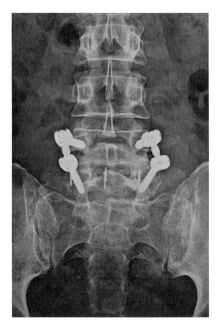

D   E

Fig. 10.2 (*continued*) **(D,E)** Postoperative lateral and anteroposterior x-rays of the lumbar spine showed good restoration of disk height and complete reduction of the spondylolisthesis with maintenance of lumbar lordosis. He experienced significant relief of his back pain and resolution of his radicular symptoms.

and foraminal height are maximally restored, indirectly decompressing the exiting nerve roots. The anterior approach avoids retraction of the neural elements and their potential injury. The ALIF also reestablishes lumbar lordosis without disrupting the posterior tension band. Its ability to restore normal lordosis is superior to TLIF.[16]

As with any fusion technique, ALIF has its disadvantages. Traversing the abdomen is accompanied by the risks of damage to abdominal viscera, great vessels, and sympathetic and lumbosacral plexus.[17] The risk of vascular injury is greatest at the L4–5 disk space. The ALIF technique also carries with it a significant risk of postoperative retrograde ejaculation in men due to injury of the superior hypogastric plexus.[18] This is an important consideration for fertility in men. The anterior exposure is accompanied by the potential for significant incisional pain, postoperative ileus, and a prolonged recovery.

A large number of studies have been published on ALIF demonstrating both efficacy and safety. Inoue et al reviewed 350 patients in 1984 who underwent ALIF at 516 levels with a 94% fusion rate and significant clinical improvement.[19] In 1998 Kuslich et al published the results of a prospective multicenter trial in which 591 patients underwent a one- or two-level ALIF. Of the 247 patients with 24-month follow-up, 93% showed evidence of successful fusion. Patients in the series also had a significant decrease in their level of pain and an improvement in their functional status.[20] Hsieh et al retrospectively evaluated 32 patients who underwent an ALIF and 25 patients who underwent TLIF over a 4-year period and compared restoration of foraminal height, local disk angle, and lumbar lordosis between the two techniques. Hsieh's study found ALIF to be superior to TLIF in all radiographic parameters, but no difference was observed in clinical outcome at 2-year follow-up.[16]

Indications for an ALIF include degenerative disk disease (DDD), grade 1–2 spondylolisthesis, and recurrent herniated nucleus pulposis (HNP). The anterior approach offers several unique advantages making it ideal for select patients. The ALIF technique allows for interbody fusion with minimal disruption of normal spinal anatomy, only disrupting the ALL, annulus, and disk, leaving the posterior tension band untouched. The anterior approach allows for placement of a large interbody graft in the anterior disk space, effectively restoring lumbar lordosis. This makes the ALIF an ideal approach for patients with significant loss of lumbar lordosis on preoperative imaging. The anterior approach may be preferred in patients with significant DDD (bone on bone) making end plate preparation difficult through alternative approaches. Patients with significant loss of posterior disk height in comparison to anterior disk height may also have superior results with an ALIF. The anterior lumbar interbody fusion is the oldest of the interbody fusion techniques, and despite the evolution of spine surgery and the development of new fusion methods, it remains a frequently utilized procedure (**Fig. 10.3**).

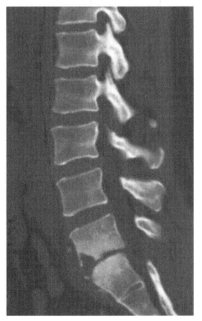
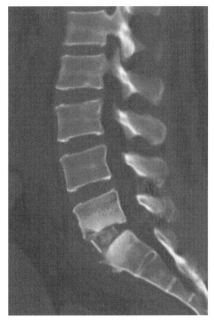

A   B

Fig. 10.3 A 37-year-old man with a history of a previous L5–S1 diskectomy, complicated by postoperative diskitis requiring debridement at an outside institution, developed chronic back and left leg pain. **(A)** Computed tomography (CT) showed significant disk space collapse at L5–S1 associated with erosion of the L5 end plate and some loss of lordosis. Surgery consisted of an L5–S1 anterior lumbar interbody fusion with percutaneous pedicle screw placement. **(B)** Postoperative CT showed satisfactory placement of a large interbody spacer with increased disk height and improved lordosis. The patient had significant relief in his back pain following surgery.

Minimally Invasive AxiaLIF with Percutaneous Pedicle Screw Stabilization

The percutaneous AxiaLIF, first described by Pimenta, is a novel minimally invasive approach for lumbar arthrodesis specifically at the L5–S1 level.[21] This technique was developed as an alternative to anterior interbody fusion techniques, which have the potential to injure the abdominal structures, and posterior fusion techniques, which can disrupt the posterior stabilizing structures.

A 15 mm incision is made 2 cm caudal to the paracoccygeal notch and the incision is advanced through the fascia. Subsequently, blunt dissection is used to confirm sufficient opening of the fascia. A guide pin/stylet is inserted and advanced under fluoroscopy and engaged on the S1–2 junction. A sharp guide pin is then inserted through S1 and into the L5–S1 disk space. A series of dilators are then used to create an osseous working channel through the sacrum. A volumetric diskectomy is performed, and bone graft material of the surgeon's preference is introduced. A titanium 3D axial rod prosthetic device is then inserted through the L5–S1 disk space and into the L5 vertebral body. This prosthetic device is composed of superior and inferior portions, each with a specific diameter and thread pitch leading to distraction of the L5–S1 interspace. The appropriate prosthesis is selected based on the degree of distraction desired. Additional bone graft and other materials can be inserted through the prosthesis prior to insertion of a threaded plug and removal of the cannula. Percutaneous pedicle screw stabilization is then performed in the usual manner to supplement the construct.[8]

The AxiaLIF technique is an approach that takes advantage of the benign fat and connective tissue occupying the presacral space. The approach avoids potential injury to the ureter, retroperitoneal structures, and great vessels. It also maintains the integrity of the musculoligamentous and bony stabilizing elements, the anterior longitudinal ligament, posterior longitudinal ligament, and annulus. This minimally disruptive approach leaves the anatomy surrounding the disk space untouched, hence minimizing iatrogenic damage to the adjacent disk level.

AxiaLIF should be avoided in patients with previous retroperitoneal surgery because there may be significant scarring along the presacral corridor increasing the potential for bowel perforation. This approach should also be avoided in patients with severe L5–S1 disk degeneration because it may be difficult to achieve the needed distraction and disk space preparation.

Given that the AxiaLIF is a relatively new approach, there is little literature on clinical outcomes. Aryan et al published a series of 35 patients treated with the AxiaLIF procedure, 25 of whom had supplemental posterior stabilization. These patients were followed for an average of 17.5 months, and 91% had radiographic evidence of fusion at last follow-up.[21]

The indications for this procedure include those pathologies requiring fusion of the L5–S1 interspace, including DDD, grade 1–2 spondylolisthesis, and recurrent disk herniations. The AxiaLIF technique is most appropriate for patients with multiple previous anterior and posterior operations that would significantly increase the risks of a repeated approach through scar tissue. The majority of patients who require an L5–S1 interbody fusion will be most appropriately managed with a minimally invasive TLIF or ALIF (**Fig. 10.4**).

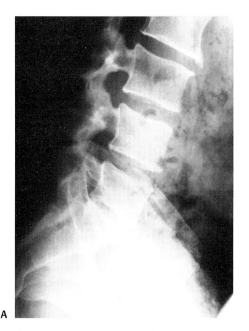

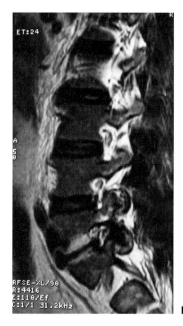

A

B

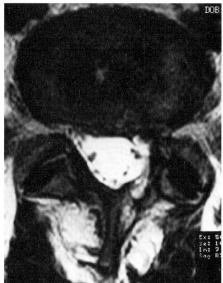

C

Fig. 10.4 A 50-year-old man with a complicated history involving three operations for disk herniations and radiculopathy at L5–S1 had intractable back and left leg pain. **(A)** Plain x-ray and **(B,C)** magnetic resonance imaging revealed L5–S1 disk space collapse and bilateral foraminal stenosis, worse on the left. Given the history of multiple posterior surgeries, an anterior approach was recommended; however, he elected not to have an anterior lumbar interbody fusion due to the associated risks but was amenable to having an AxiaLIF (TranS1, Wilmington, NC). (*continued*)

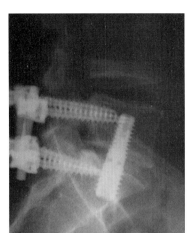
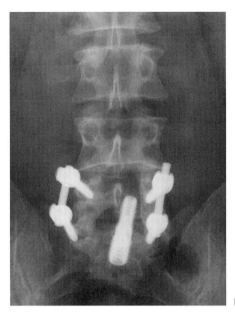

D · E

Fig. 10.4 (*continued*) **(D,E)** Postoperative imaging revealed satisfactory placement of the interbody device with increased disk height. The patient had complete resolution of his back pain with significant relief in his radicular symptoms.

◆ Discussion

At the L4–5 level and above the surgeon can perform one of three interbody fusion techniques in a minimally invasive manner. The patient without an antecedent history of extensive abdominal surgery with a low-grade spondylolisthesis or significant degenerative disk disease with foraminal stenosis, in the absence of severe canal stenosis, is an ideal candidate for a lateral interbody fusion with posterior stabilization. An ALIF can also be performed in this clinical scenario, although the risks become greater to the retroperitoneal vessels as the pathology ascends the lumbar spine. In a patient with severe canal stenosis or lateral recess stenosis from a disk herniation, a minimally invasive TLIF affords the ability to directly decompress the neural elements within the canal via an ipsilateral foraminotomy or bilateral decompressive laminectomy. In patients with severe DDD with significant collapse or loss of lordosis, ALIF may provide superior results. ALIF allows access to the anterior disk space, the ability to distract, and the shortest operative distance, which, in the setting of difficult disk space preparation, are all critical advantages. ALIF also allows for placement of a large interbody graft in the anterior disk space, allowing for superior restoration of lumbar lordosis and overall sagittal balance. ALIF may also prove to be the better approach in patients with significant posterior disk space collapse in comparison with the anterior disk space.

At the L5–S1 disk space, the surgeon again has three minimally invasive approaches for lumbar arthrodesis because the lateral interbody techniques cannot be performed at this level. As discussed previously, patients with concurrent severe foraminal stenosis or lumbar canal stenosis may be best served with a minimally invasive TLIF. In cases of severe DDD (bone on bone) or significant posterior disk space collapse, ALIF may be the most appropriate approach. AxiaLIF remains a procedure indicated for a very select group of patients with contraindications to the minimally invasive TLIF or ALIF.

In patients with previous operations, it is often best to avoid associated scar tissue because this significantly increases the potential for complications. In patients with previous posterior spinal surgery, the lateral interbody fusion may prove to be the ideal technique, given that it provides the surgeon with a corridor of virgin tissue for spinal access. The TLIF technique may also be an option in these patients because the posterolateral trajectory from a paramedian starting point through naive tissue often avoids the majority of scarring, although there remains the potential for scar tissue in the epidural space. In patients with previous abdominal operations it is often best to avoid an anterior approach, including the ALIF and AxiaLIF. The XLIF approach may also prove to be difficult depending on the degree of retroperitoneal scarring from previous operations.

Spine surgeons have a choice of several interbody fusion techniques for the management of lumbar mechanical back pain, radicular pain, recurrent HNP, and instability. Many of these procedures can be done in a minimally disruptive fashion in an effort to reduce morbidity and maximize preservation of normal spinal anatomy. It is imperative that we understand the advantages, disadvantages, and appropriate indications for these procedures so that we are able to fashion the ideal surgical procedure for each individual patient.

References

1. Fritzell P, Hägg O, Wessberg P, Nordwall A; Swedish Lumbar Spine Study Group. 2001 Volvo Award Winner in Clinical Studies: Lumbar fusion versus nonsurgical treatment for chronic low back pain: a multicenter randomized controlled trial from the Swedish Lumbar Spine Study Group. Spine (Phila Pa 1976) 2001;26:2521–2532

2. Albee FH. Transplantation of a portion of the tibia into the spine for Pott's disease: a preliminary report. JAMA 1911;57:885–886

3. Hibbs RH. An operation for progressive spinal deformities. New York Med J 1911;93:1013–1016

4. First Description of Lumbar Interbody Fusion published by Capener and Colleagues

5. Cloward RB. The treatment of ruptured lumbar intervertebral discs by vertebral body fusion, I: Indications, operative technique, after care. J Neurosurg 1953;10:154–168

6. Harms JG, Jeszensky D. The unilateral, transforaminal approach for the posterior lumbar interbody fusion. Oper Orthop Traumatol 1998;6:88–99

7. Ozgur BM, Aryan HE, Pimenta L, Taylor WR. Extreme lateral interbody fusion (XLIF): a novel surgical technique for anterior lumbar interbody fusion. Spine J 2006;6:435–443

8. Marotta N, Cosar M, Pimenta L, Khoo LT. A novel minimally invasive presacral approach and instrumentation technique for anterior L5-S1 intervertebral discectomy and fusion: technical description and case presentations. Neurosurg Focus 2006;20:E9

9. Tay BBK, Berven S. Indications, techniques, and complications of lumbar interbody fusion. Semin Neurol 2002;22:221–230

10. Foley KT, Holly LT, Schwender JD. Minimally invasive lumbar fusion. Spine (Phila Pa 1976) 2003;28(15, Suppl):S26–S35

11. Holley LT, Schwender JD, Rouben DP, Foley KT. Minimally invasive transforaminal lumbar interbody fusion: indications, techniques and complications. Neurosurg Focus 2006;20: E6

12. Lowe TG, Tahernia AD, O'Brien MF, Smith DAB. Unilateral transforaminal posterior lumbar interbody fusion (TLIF): indications, technique, and 2-year results. J Spinal Disord Tech 2002;15:31–38

13. Schwender JD, Holly LT, Rouben DP, Foley KT. Minimally invasive transforaminal lumbar interbody fusion (TLIF): technical feasibility and initial results. J Spinal Disord Tech 2005;18(Suppl):S1–S6

14. Jang JS, Lee SH. Minimally invasive transforaminal lumbar interbody fusion with ipsilateral pedicle screw and contralateral facet screw fixation. J Neurosurg Spine 2005;3:218–223

15. Ozgur BM, Aryan HE, Pimenta L, Taylor WR. Extreme lateral interbody fusion (XLIF): a novel surgical technique for anterior lumbar interbody fusion. Spine J 2006;6:435–443

16. Hsieh PC, Koski TR, O'Shaughnessy BA, et al. Anterior lumbar interbody fusion in comparison with transforaminal lumbar interbody fusion: implications for the restoration of foraminal height, local disc angle, lumbar lordosis, and sagittal balance. J Neurosurg Spine 2007;7:379–386

17. Rauzzino MJ, Shaffrey CI, Nockels RP, Wiggins GC, Rock J, Wagner J. Anterior lumbar fusion with titanium threaded and mesh interbody cages. Neurosurg Focus 1999;7:e7

18. Sasso RC, Kenneth Burkus J, LeHuec JC. Retrograde ejaculation after anterior lumbar interbody fusion: transperitoneal versus retroperitoneal exposure. Spine (Phila Pa 1976) 2003;28:1023–1026

19. Inoue SI, Watanabe T, Hirose A, et al. Anterior discectomy and interbody fusion for lumbar disc herniation: a review of 350 cases. Clin Orthop Relat Res 1984;183:22–31

20. Kuslich SD, Ulstrom CL, Griffith SL, Ahern JW, Dowdle JD. The Bagby and Kuslich method of lumbar interbody fusion: history, techniques, and 2-year follow-up results of a United States prospective, multicenter trial. Spine (Phila Pa 1976) 1998;23:1267–1278

21. Marotta N, Cosar M, Pimenta L, Khoo LT. A novel minimally invasive presacral approach and instrumentation technique for anterior L5-S1 intervertebral discectomy and fusion: technical description and case presentations. Neurosurg Focus 2006;20:E9

22. Aryan HE, Newman CB, Gold JJ, Acosta FL Jr, Coover C, Ames CP. Percutaneous axial lumbar interbody fusion (AxiaLIF) of the L5–S1 segment: initial clinical and radiographic experience. Minim Invasive Neurosurg 2008;51:225–230

Section IV

Other Considerations

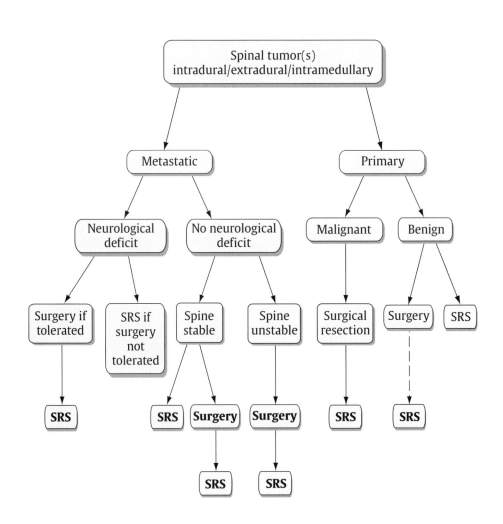

11

Stereotactic Spinal Radiosurgery for Primary and Metastatic Disease

Edward A. Monaco III and Peter C. Gerszten

Tumors of the spine and spinal elements result in a considerable amount of morbidity. Primary tumors of the spine are relatively rare, but when present frequently cause symptoms and historically have proven very difficult to treat.[1] Metastatic disease is severalfold more frequent. Nearly 200,000 cases of spinal metastases are identified in North America each year.[1-3] Some 10% of these can be expected to result in neural element compression. In the setting of better multimodality treatment for cancer and improved long-term survival for its sufferers, it is likely that these numbers will only grow in the future. Therefore, it is becoming ever more important for clinicians to be well versed in the diagnosis and management of spinal tumors.

The goals for the treatment of spinal tumors are several and include the following: prevention of local disease progression, preservation of spinal structural stability, preservation of neurological function, and the abolishment of pain.[4] Traditionally, achieving these goals has involved treatment by surgery, radiation therapy, or chemotherapy, alone or in some combination.[5] Over the last 2 decades, clinicians have become acutely aware of the benefits of applying the concept of minimal invasiveness to these modalities to offer maximum treatment effect with the least adverse sequelae. Whether molecularly targeting a specific kinase cascade or applying minimally invasive surgical techniques, attempts at the preservation of unaffected normal tissues are clearly advantageous.

A similar paradigm has been applied to the field of spinal radiotherapy. Conventional radiation therapy, the delivery of one or two low-precision and nonconformal radiation beams, is a well-established treatment modality for malignancies of the spine and is often the initial approach taken.[5-11] Unfortunately, the effectiveness of conventional radiation therapy to the spine is limited by the relative intolerance of certain surrounding tissues to high doses of radiation, in particular the spinal cord and other neural elements. Thus treatment doses far below the optimal therapeutic doses are applied, resulting in frequent recurrence or progression of disease due to an insufficient radiobiological effect.[12–14]

In contrast, the precise application of a tightly confined radiation dose to the desired treatment area, as has been the well-documented experience for intracranial stereotactic radiosurgery, should serve to allow for targeted optimal dosing, better tumor and symptom control, with a greatly reduced likelihood of injury to adjacent normal tissue structures.[12,15–23] With the advent of improved imaging techniques, advances in radiation delivery, and computerized treatment planning, stereotactic spinal radiosurgery has become a valuable tool for the treatment of selected patients with both primary and metastatic tumors of the spine.

◆ Background of Stereotactic Spinal Radiosurgery

Radiosurgery can be defined as the precise delivery of a highly conformal, large radiation dose to a specific target via a stereotactic approach.[24] Spinal radiosurgery draws its origins from the use of radiosurgery for the treatment of benign and malignant intracranial disease.[25–30] Conventional intracranial radiosurgery utilizes a frame-based system that requires the application of a rigid frame to the skull for immobilization and localization of the target lesion in space. Intracranial radiosurgery is feasible because lesions within the skull have a fixed relationship in space to the skull itself. Therefore, with a rigidly applied stereotactic frame serving as a fiducial reference system, the accurate targeting and delivery of a radiation dose via multiple beams is possible. Single-fraction, high-dose treatments have thus become a favorable methodology. This technique has proven an extremely effective tool for the control of pathologies ranging from meningiomas to brain metastases.

Within the spine, lesions can have a specific fixed relationship in space to one or more vertebral segments. In contrast to the cranial vault, however, the spine is a highly mobile structure. Thus, to parallel intracranial radiosurgery with spinal radiosurgery, rigid immobilization of the spine near the target lesion with a stereotactic frame would be required. Early efforts utilized such invasive rigid external frames placed directly on the spine (i.e., the Hamilton-Lulu extracranial stereotactic frame), but these have not generally been adopted.[31,32] An early alternative was the Lax extracranial stereotactic frame that utilized noninvasive immobilization with a vacuum pillow or foam pad within a computed tomographically (CT) detectable frame covering the patient from the head down to the midthigh.[33,34]

Since the first suggestion of using linear-accelerator (LINAC) based stereotactic spinal radiosurgery in the mid-1990s, the delivery of highly conformal high-dose radiation to spinal disease has been pursued by several centers.[1,12,14,16–18,21,22,24,35–44] Moreover, spinal radiosurgery for primary and metastatic tumors has more recently demonstrated safety and efficacy.[12,14,16,17,21,22,24,36,38–40,42,44] Improved imaging techniques for treatment planning and localization, combined with the advent of intensity-modulated radiation therapy (IMRT), allow clinicians to treat lesions anywhere from the paraspinal area to intramedullary locations with high target dose confirmation and sparing of normal tissues.

◆ Spinal Cord Tolerance

Highly conformal target dosing to the spine provides the theoretical advantage of greatly limiting the likelihood of radiation myelitis. Despite an extensive experience with spinal radiation, little is known clinically regarding the tolerance of the human spinal cord to large single-fraction doses.[22,45,46] Thus, the basis for our understanding regarding cord tolerance is derived from series in which external beam radiation was used and the entire thickness of the cord was irradiated. The total doses (TD) at which there is a 5% probability of radiation myelitis after 5 years for 5–20 cm lengths of spinal cord has been estimated to be 5 Gy.[47] These conclusions are extrapolated from data produced in the 1940s. Despite this, these estimations have been adopted widely by those administering spinal radiation. Thus, to decrease the risk of spinal cord necrosis, standard fractionation schemes have stated cord tolerance to be 45 to 50 Gy. A common fractionation scheme of 1.8 to 2 Gy per fraction for a total of 45 to 50 Gy falls within the radiation tolerance of the spinal cord. Doses of 8 Gy in a single fraction have been delivered to long portions of the spinal cord without reported myelopathy.[48,49]

One study of 172 patients receiving fractionated radiation therapy to cervical and thoracic segments reported nine cases of radiation-induced myelopathy with a fractionation schedule of 40 to 70 Gy over 2 to 3 weeks.[50] Another series of 387 patients receiving large single-fraction treatments for bronchial carcinoma had 17 patients suffer radiation myelitis.[51] The average total dose for these patients was 38 Gy. Of 109 patient receiving fractionated regimens of 57 to 62 Gy for head and neck cancers, seven developed myelopathy.[7] Eight of 203 cases developed radiation myelitis in another series where patients were treated with a total dose of 54 to 60 Gy to the cervical and thoracic spine.[52] Only one of another 652 patients, all of whom received standard fractionation total doses greater than 60 Gy, showed evidence of myelitis.[53] Finally, of 350 patients treated with a total radiation dose of 33 to 43.5 Gy for chest tumors, three cases of radiation myelitis were reported.[54]

◆ Treatment Planning and Dosing

A spinal radiosurgery procedure can be divided into four unique components. First, the patient must be immobilized and/or have fiducials implanted for image guidance. Second, CT imaging is performed for treatment planning and generation of digitally reconstructed radiographs (DRRs). Third, the radiation dose planning is completed. Finally, the actual radiation dose is delivered to the patient. Completion of these tasks involves a team of individuals including a surgeon, a radiation oncologist, and a medical physicist. Spinal radiosurgery is usually performed in an outpatient setting.

Treatment prescription involves a combination of volume and dose quantifications. The clinical target volume (CTV) includes the gross tumor volume (GTV) and any adjacent areas interpreted as having a high likelihood of tumor involvement. Both the CTV and all the structures for which it is critical to avoid toxic radiation dosing are identified during planning. This can be done by outlining the lesion (GTV) from CT or magnetic resonance imaging (MRI) fusion capability. Dosing is also determined on the basis of tumor histology and previous radiation exposure to normal tissues, especially the spinal cord. However, to date, little or no published data are available that provide guidelines for the most efficacious and least toxic dosing schedules. Dosing and fractionation schedules vary widely. It has been the practice at the University of Pittsburgh to apply a single-fraction radiosurgery paradigm on the basis of the large experience with the Leksell Gamma Knife (Elekta, Inc., Norcross, GA) for intracranial disease.

A tumor dose maintained at 12 to 20 Gy to the 80% isodose line contoured to the edge of the target volume is used for single-fraction therapy. This provides a maximum intratumoral dose ranging from 15 to 30 Gy. Sixteen Gy to the tumor margin with a maximum intratumoral dose of 20 Gy has demonstrated excellent tumor control with minimal risk of radiation toxicity to the spinal cord or cauda equina.[38] Other dosing schedules have been reported with 6 to 30 Gy in 1 to 5 fractions.[12,17,18,22,23,55–58]

During treatment planning, the spinal cord and/or cauda equina are outlined as critical structures. From the cauda equina distally, the entire spinal canal is outlined. For single-fraction schemes, the recommended maximum spinal cord dose is below 10 Gy to avoid the possibility of radiation-induced myelitis. A dose of up to 14 Gy appears to be a safe maximum dose to the cauda equina.[46] The aforementioned constraints are applied together with the target dose prescription during treatment planning. To accomplish this, the treatment team uses the desired dose distribution and applies inverse treatment planning to design a field setup (beam angles) and appropriate beam intensities.

◆ Image Guidance and Treatment Conformality

Two principles required for successful radiosurgery are those of target localization and target immobilization. Precise patient setup and lesion localization are critical for the execution of a radiosurgery treatment, and various methodologies have been utilized to position and immobilize patients.[1,48] One paradigm mirrors that of intracranial radiosurgery and involves the placement of a rigidly fixed frame in which the patient undergoes CT imaging and ultimately treatment.[40] Subsequently, success has been achieved with frameless techniques.

One approach for spinal radiosurgery has been to immobilize the patient in a noninvasive stereotactic body frame or immobilization cradle. These devices do not ensure that the patient will remain perfectly positioned, but by obtaining pre- and posttreatment imaging, acceptable immobilization results have been obtained for devices using this technique. One example of this is the near-simultaneous CT image-guided stereotactic radiotherapy system at MD Anderson Cancer Center. This system integrates a CT-on-rails scanner with a linear accelerator. Each patient is immobilized in a moldable body cushion vacuum wrapped with a plastic fixation sheet. Patients are transferred directly from the CT scanner to the linear accelerator couch via a rail system.[23] Another example is the Memorial Stereotactic Body Frame (MSBF), developed at Memorial Sloan Kettering. The patient is externally immobilized with a series of pressure plates and has CT images obtained on a scanner in the same room as the linear accelerator. This pretreatment CT is automatically registered with the planning CT using bony landmarks. A second registration of the fiducial system in the treatment and planning scans allows positioning error in the body frame to be determined. Final positioning verification is completed through comparison of the cone beam CT, orthogonal portal images, and digitally reconstructed radiographs from the initial planning CT.[57]

A second approach involves the frequent acquisition of localizing images during the actual treatment and adjusting the patient's position accordingly. The CyberKnife Image-Guided Radiosurgery System (Accuray, Inc., Sunnyvale, CA) exemplifies this approach. The CyberKnife system consists of a 6 megavolt (mV) compact linear accelerator mounted on a computer-controlled, six-axis robotic manipulator, and two orthogonally positioned diagnostic x-ray cameras.[59,60] Images from the x-ray cameras are acquired and processed to identify radiographic features. They are then automatically compared with the planning CT so that precise tumor position is communicated via a real-time control loop to the robotic manipulator that aligns the radiation beam with the planned target.[39,61–63] No additional immobilization is required other than the treatment couch because the positions of the bony structures are checked numerous times during treatment. As a result, any changes in tumor position are quickly detected and corrected during the course of treatment.[1]

Radiation delivery for radiosurgery requires precisely shaped beams. This is accomplished in part via 360 degree rotatable gantries to allow for multiple beam directions. Beam angles are selected to provide the ideal coverage of the target volume while sparing normal tissues. The beams can be further modified by the use of collimators that can attenuate the beam and precisely define the treatment field. A multileaf collimator (MLC) continuously adjusts the field size as the beams are shaped through movements of its leaves. For radiosurgery, the leaves are very small, allowing for accurate delivery of radiation to extremely small field sizes (micro MLC). The concept is referred to as intensity-modulated radiotherapy (IMRT).

The Novalis Shaped-Beam Surgery unit (BrainLAB, Westchester, IL) is an example of this approach to spinal radiosurgery. It is a specialized treatment device consisting of a 6 mV linear accelerator equipped with a micro MLC and dual in-room kilovoltage (keV) x-ray units. Two digitally reconstructed radiographs are generated from the simulation CT scan at the same orientation as the x-ray images. The system then compares the internal anatomy noted on the x-rays with that of the digitally reconstructed images and automatically adjusts the patient position based on isocenter deviations.[56]

The ability to acquire volumetric or three-dimensional pretreatment imaging has improved treatment accuracy and precision, and it allows for the detection of rotational errors in patient setup and enables robust automatic registration procedures. The TomoTherapy Hi-Art system (TomoTherapy, Inc., Madison, WI) integrates treatment planning and CT-based image-guided helical IMRT.[35,64] It consists of a small 6 meV linear accelerator that has been mounted directly upon a CT scanner gantry. A 64-multileaf collimator modulates the beam output, making this device capable of delivering highly conformal radiation doses to multiple targets simultaneously. Finally, daily pretreatment megavolt CT scans can be co-registered with the planning CT scan to ensure accurate patient setup.

Cone beam imaging uses a gantry-mounted kilovolt source and detector that can acquire several hundred projection images with each full gantry rotation. These images can be converted into CT-like axial slices via image reconstruction software. Cone beam scans provide high spatial resolution of bony and soft tissue structures, thus allowing for the setup of sites with submillimeter targeting errors.[1] The Elekta Synergy S (Elekta, Inc., Atlanta, GA) was the first digitally controlled linear accelerator for image-guided radiotherapy enabling the acquisition of three-dimensional images at the time of treatment with the patient in the treatment position. The device's robotic couch responds to detected errors in setup by making adjustments in the patient's position, thus ensuring accurate radiation targeting. The Novalis TX device (Varian Medical Systems, Palo Alto, CA and BrainLAB, Westchester, IL) incorporates cone beam imaging with dual in-room x-ray units.

◆ Radiosurgery for Metastatic Spinal Disease

Similar to the pattern with intracranial radiosurgery in the past decade, the indications for spinal radiosurgery are evolving as clinical experience increases with this new technology (**Figs. 11.1** and **11.2**). Lesions can be of nearly any histological type and can be located anywhere along the spine, both extradural and intradural. Candidate tumors may be those for which a surgical resection would be too morbid, or for those with a residual component that could not be excised. Candidate patients may be too ill to tolerate a surgical procedure or may have a life expectancy too short to make surgery a reasonable option. Radiosurgery can be used to prevent tumor progression that could lead to spinal instability or neural element compromise. Indeed, spinal radiosurgery, like that for intracranial radiosurgery, can be the primary treatment modality and prevent the necessity of re-irradiation by improving initial tumor control.

Pain

Pain is the primary indication for the treatment of spinal tumors in a substantial proportion of cases. Historically, radiation has proven an effective way to treat pain in the setting of spinal malignancies. Unfortunately, conventional external beam radiotherapy may provide less pain relief because it is limited in its dosing by the limited tolerance of adjacent tissues. In one large series of spine radiosurgery in 435 cases from our institution, 86% of patients had overall long-term pain improvement, the specific results of which depended on tumor histology. Ninety-six percent of breast cancer patients, 96% of melanoma patients, 94% of renal cell carcinoma patients, and 93% of patients with lung cancer experienced durable pain relief.[65–68] Pain relief, however, is not immediate and often occurs from days to weeks following the procedure. Radiosurgery is also efficacious for radicular pain caused by tumor-mediated nerve root compression.

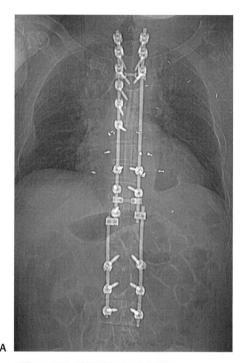

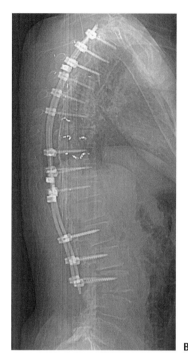

A

B

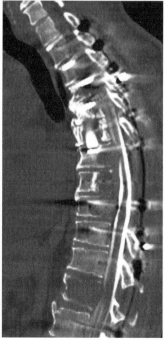

C

Fig 11.1 Case example of a 50-year-old man with metastatic thyroid carcinoma. **(A)** AP and **(B)** lateral x-rays of a patient who had previously undergone an open surgical decompression and instrumented fusion from T2 to L3, skipping the diseased level of T12. The patient had undergone prior conventional fractionated radiotherapy to the T12 level. **(C)** Follow-up imaging revealed radiographic progression of tumor with spinal cord compression at T12. It was felt that radiosurgery was indicated to avoid a major open surgical intervention in the middle of the prior long construct. For the radiosurgery treatment, the prescribed radiation dose to the gross tumor volume was 18 Gy to be delivered using nine co-planar beams in a single fraction (Synergy S, Elekta Inc., Atlanta, GA). (*continued*)

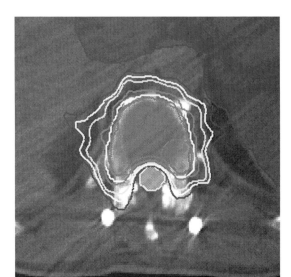

D

E

Fig 11.1 (*continued*)   Case example of a 50-year-old man with metastatic thyroid carcinoma. (D) Axial and (E) sagittal images of the treatment plan. The gross tumor volume was 39.9 cm³, and the spinal cord received a maximum dose of 11 Gy. Less than 1.0 cm³ of the spinal cord received greater than 8 Gy.

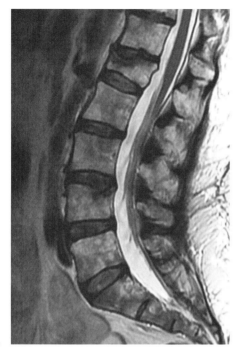

Fig. 11.2 Case example of a 54-year-old woman with metastatic breast cancer. The patient had previously undergone conventional fractionated radiotherapy to her lumbar spine. She was referred for neurosurgical consultation with the complaint of severe lower back pain. **(A)** Magnetic resonance imaging revealed compression fractures at L1 and L4 with disease progression at L1, L3, and L4. She was felt to be a candidate for percutaneous methylmethacrylate augmentation followed by radiosurgery. (*continued*)

A

The Georgetown University Hospital experience is the largest to date regarding data on pain control and quality of life improvement.[19,58] Following radiosurgery with a follow-up period of up to 24 months, patients experienced a statistically significant improvement in pain control and maintenance of quality of life. Adverse events were infrequent and minor. Ninety percent of patients treated by the Memorial Sloan Kettering group, with a median follow-up of 12 months, experienced excellent palliation of symptoms.[1] Several other series report similar efficacy for pain control.[12,14,16,18,21,22,69]

Radiographic Tumor Progression

Current treatment paradigms for spinal malignancies often involve conventional radiation therapy and/or surgery. If these approaches fail and tumor progression is detected radiographically, further conventional radiation therapy is precluded due to the likelihood of spinal cord toxicity. Radiosurgery is often used in this "salvage" situation.

At the University of Pittsburgh, 88% of cases in a series of 500 with progressive spinal disease showed long-term radiographic tumor control.[38] As with pain, the extent of tumor control depended on histology: breast (100%), lung (100%), renal cell (87%), and melanoma (75%). The group at Memorial Sloan Kettering reported a 90% long-term radiographic control rate.[1] Several groups have reported similar radiographic control rates for radiosurgery following tumor progression.[12,14,17,18,58,70]

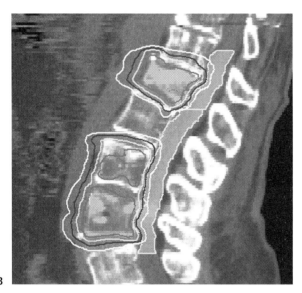

Fig. 11.2 (*continued*)   **(B)** Sagittal and **(C)** axial images of the treatment plan. For the radiosurgery treatment, the prescribed radiation dose to the gross tumor volume was 16 Gy to be delivered using nine co-planar beams in a single fraction (Synergy S, Elekta Inc., Atlanta, GA). The gross tumor volume was 68.3 cm³, and the cauda equina received a maximum dose of 11 Gy.

Primary Treatment Modality

If the evolution of spinal radiosurgery follows that of intracranial radiosurgery, it is likely that radiosurgery will become an upfront treatment for certain cases of spinal malignancies. For instance, in patients with one symptomatic lesion, yet numerous radiographic ones, primary spinal radiosurgery offers several benefits. First, upfront radiosurgery greatly decreases radiation dose to the neural elements and other normal tissue, which permits future repeat radiosurgery. It avoids vertebral radiation-induced myelosuppression, thus permitting better systemic therapy. Treatment can be delivered in possibly a single session with a radiobiologically larger dose than can be delivered by conventional fractionated radiation therapy. With an upfront approach, long-term tumor control has been demonstrated by our group in 90% of cases, again depending on histology (100% control rate in breast, lung, and renal cell, with 75% control of melanoma metastases).[38,65,68]

After Open Surgery or Boost

Often, residual tumor is or must be left behind following open surgery. This is especially true when malignancy is widespread and the primary indication for surgery is neural element decompression. Thus surgery can be undertaken and spinal instrumentation placed to stabilize as necessary, with spinal radiosurgery following at a later time to treat the residual disease. Moreover, the potential to treat with radiosurgery can alter the surgical plan. For instance, less severely affected adjacent levels may not require open surgery, but instead can be treated with radiosurgery. This could decrease surgical morbidity by limiting the operative duration and complexity. Finally, unlike standard radiation therapy, radiosurgery can be performed shortly after surgery. Given the negligible dose delivered to the subcutaneous layer and fascia, radiosurgery can be given within days, instead of weeks, after open surgery. The steep fall-off of the radiation dose prevents excessive skin exposure and limits the danger of wound failure.

Evaluation of adjuvant spinal radiosurgery following open surgery has been shown to be a successful treatment algorithm with associated disease stabilization and the potential for improving neurological function.[70] As with the University of Pittsburgh experience with intracranial radiosurgery, we have observed that the combination of open surgery followed by spinal radiosurgery to the residual tumor bed can be a very safe as well as effective therapy.[38]

When highly radioresistant tumors necessitate treatment (e.g., renal cell carcinoma, sarcoma, melanoma) radiosurgery can serve as a boost therapy to conventional radiation. Emphasis is again on the fact that the radiosurgical treatment limits exposure to surrounding normal tissues while providing large radiobiological doses to the tumor. Published series have shown this "boost" paradigm to be an effective method of providing excellent long-term radiographic tumor control.[1,22]

Progressive Neurological Deficit

In the setting of progressive neurological deficit, open surgical decompression has been the mainstay of treatment. However, there are cases in which open surgery is relatively contraindicated and the risks are too great. Historically, conventional radiation therapy has been applied to these symptomatic lesions. In the University of Pittsburgh experience, for patients in whom open surgery was contraindicated, 86% of 42 patients experienced some clinical improvement in neurological deficits.[38] Similar results have been published with other series.[1,58]

◆ Radiosurgery for Primary Malignant Spinal Disease

Primary tumors of the spine are severalfold less frequent than metastatic disease. The most common primary tumors of the spinal column include chordoma, chondrosarcoma, and osteogenic sarcoma. Unfortunately, most primary histologies are relatively radioresistant, and the limited doses of conventional radiation that can be applied to avoid spinal cord toxicity are not sufficient to yield successful long-term tumor control. Indeed, it is the lower-dose areas of the radiation field that most likely result in tumor recurrence. From a radiobiological perspective, larger fraction sizes yield better tumor control for such tumors. However, given the great difficulty in producing complete surgical resections of primary tumors, radiation is a critical adjunctive therapy. To increase the radiation dose to primary lesions and spare normal tissues, spinal radiosurgery is among the radiation techniques that are being evaluated.[71] To date, however, few published data are available regarding the efficacy of spinal radiosurgery for primary spine tumors.

◆ Radiosurgery for Primary Benign Spinal Disease

Experience with the treatment of benign spinal disease via radiosurgery is also less extensive than that for metastatic tumors. Benign intradural extramedullary tumors and arteriovenous malformations are two areas of focus. Again, this closely parallels the evolution of intracranial radiosurgery.

The current initial treatment algorithm for spinal meningiomas, schwannomas, and neurofibromas is that of microsurgical resection. By definition, they are intradural and often intimately associated with the normal neural structures, making a safe radiosurgery dose delivery problematic. These tumors tend not to be infiltrative, and when they are totally resected, cure can be achieved.[72,73] Indications for radiosurgical treatment of these tumors parallel those for metastatic disease. Patients in whom an open surgery is contraindicated are potential candidates.[74] For circumstances like neurocutaneous syndromes in which many lesions, even many symptomatic lesions, may be present, radiosurgery is a viable treatment option. Finally, in the presence of tumor recurrence where repeat open surgery is made more difficult and cure is less likely, minimally invasive radiosurgery could be useful.[74]

At the University of Pittsburgh, we have seen excellent results treating benign intradural extramedullary tumors with radiosurgery, mirroring the findings of intracranial radiosurgery. In our series of more than 100 tumors, more than 70% of patients had durable pain improvement, and excellent long-term radiographic tumor control was observed.[75] Long-term radiographic response has also been demonstrated.[74] One theoretical risk of radiosurgery for benign tumors is that of secondary malignant transformation. However, no such case has been reported to date.

Meningiomas

Meningiomas are derived from arachnoid cap cells, have a female predominance, and are found most frequently in the thoracic spine. In one series, treatment of 16 tumors by CyberKnife resulted in two thirds of them being radiographically stabilized and one third showing a decrease in their radiographic tumor size.[74] Many of these patients also derived discernible improvements in pain level and strength. We have treated 13 spinal meningiomas, all with a single-fraction paradigm as an adjunct to open surgery. Radiographic tumor control was 100% with a median follow-up of 17 months.[75]

Neurofibromas

Neurofibromas of the spine are commonly associated with neurofibromatosis type 1 (NF1). The lesions predominate in the cervical spine, and they tend to be multiple. In a series of seven patients with nine neurofibromas treated by radiosurgery, 86% demonstrated radiographic tumor control.[74] However, symptom improvement did not correspond with tumor stabilization. In the 25 neurofibroma cases treated with radiosurgery at the University of Pittsburgh (NF1, 21 cases; NF2, four cases), radiographic tumor progression was absent.[75] However, only eight of the 13 patients treated for pain symptoms experienced pain relief. Interestingly, the patients who failed to experience pain relief all had NF1, paralleling the aforementioned report and suggesting the NF1-associated neurofibromas may be less responsive to radiosurgery. This may correspond with the observation of poorer microsurgical results for the treatment of neurofibromas in patients with NF1. The reason for this unusual behavior is not yet known. Perhaps the more infiltrative nature of NF1 neurofibromas results in nerve injury that is not reversible with tumor stabilization by radiosurgery.

Schwannomas

Schwannomas are the most common benign intradural extramedullary tumor of the spine.[76] They appear with equal frequency in all locations of the spine. In one series of 30 schwannomas treated with radiosurgery, all but one patient had radiographic tumor control.[74] One third of patients experienced symptom improvement, but nearly 20% had a clinical decline after treatment. The University of Pittsburgh experience includes the treatment of 35 schwannomas. Eighty-two percent (14 of 17) of patients had significant pain improvement.[75] Six of seven patients treated primarily with radiosurgery demonstrated radiographic tumor control. Three patients required subsequent surgical resection for new or persistent neurological deficits.

Arteriovenous Malformations

Stereotactic radiosurgery for cerebral arteriovenous malformations (AVMs) has proven a highly efficacious and minimally invasive therapy.[77] For lesions 2.5 cm or smaller, obliteration rates of 80 to 85% have often been reported.[37,78–82] Following radiosurgery, gradual hyperplasia of the AVMs' nidal arteries ensues, ultimately leading to their closure.[83] These results suggest the utility of spinal radiosurgery in treating spinal AVMs. Indeed, spinal AVMs have been successfully treated with radiosurgery.[84] There are several subtypes of spinal AVMs; however, those with a relatively compact nidus would represent optimal targets. Type II spinal cord AVMs, or glomus AVMs, possess a compact vascular nidus. They have proven historically difficult to treat with traditional microsurgical and endovascular approaches and were often left untreated.

The Stanford series of 23 patients with spinal cord AVMs treated with CyberKnife technology is the largest series reported.[85] Twenty-two of these AVMs were deemed to be type II in classification. Twelve were located in the cervical spine, eight in the thoracic spine, and three in the conus region. The range of marginal doses was 16 to 21 Gy (20.3 Gy mean) over one to four sessions. Although postoperative MRI demonstrated reduced AVM size, only eight patients underwent spinal angiograms. Of these eight, three were found to have complete angiographic obliteration. No subsequent rebleeding events were noted with a mean follow-up of 35 months. This limited experience, however, dictates that the future of radiosurgery for the treatment of spinal AVMs remains undetermined.

◆ Conclusion

The indications for spinal radiosurgery are evolving. Radiosurgery offers a minimally invasive and highly efficacious approach for the treatment of both primary and metastatic tumors of the spine. It avoids much of the morbidity associated with open surgery, even minimally invasive open surgery. Moreover, the ability to successfully treat malignant lesions of the spine with radiosurgery can radically alter the extent of open surgery. Radiation exposure to large segments of the spinal cord and normal tissues can be significantly minimized. As such, much larger radiobiological doses can be delivered compared with conventional fractionated external beam radiotherapy. Indeed, as more is learned, radiosurgery as a primary treatment modality is likely to become ever more commonplace, just as it has become for intracranial malignancies.

References

1. Yamada Y, Lovelock DM, Bilsky MH. A review of image-guided intensity-modulated radiotherapy for spinal tumors. Neurosurgery 2007;61:226–235
2. Black P. Spinal metastasis: current status and recommended guidelines for management. Neurosurgery 1979;5:726–746
3. Gokaslan ZL, York JE, Walsh GL, et al. Transthoracic vertebrectomy for metastatic spinal tumors. J Neurosurg 1998;89:599–609
4. Lu C, Stomper PC, Drislane FW, et al. Suspected spinal cord compression in breast cancer patients: a multidisciplinary risk assessment. Breast Cancer Res Treat 1998;51:121–131
5. Gerszten PC, Welch WC. Current surgical management of metastatic spinal disease. Oncology (Williston Park) 2000;14:1013–1024
6. Faul CM, Flickinger JC. The use of radiation in the management of spinal metastases. J Neurooncol 1995;23:149–161
7. Kim YH, Fayos JV. Radiation tolerance of the cervical spinal cord. Radiology 1981;139:473–478
8. Markoe AM, Schwade JG. The role of radiation therapy in the management of spine and spinal cord tumors. In: Rea GL, ed. Spine Tumors. Park Ridge, IL: American Association of Neurological Surgeons; 1994:23–35
9. Shapiro W, Posner JB. Medical vs surgical treatment of metastatic spinal cord tumors. In: Thompson R, Green J, eds. Controversies in Neurology. New York: Raven Press; 1983:57
10. Sundaresan N, Digiacinto GV, Hughes JEO, Cafferty M, Vallejo A. Treatment of neoplastic spinal cord compression: results of a prospective study. Neurosurgery 1991;29:645–650
11. Sundaresan N, Krol G, Digiacinto CV, et al. Metastatic tumors of the spine. In: Sundaresan B, Schmidek H, Schiller A, et al, eds. Tumors of the Spine. Philadelphia, PA: WB Saunders; 1990:279

12. De Salles AA, Pedroso AG, Medin P, et al. Spinal lesions treated with Novalis shaped beam intensity-modulated radiosurgery and stereotactic radiotherapy. J Neurosurg 2004;101(Suppl 3):435–440

13. Loblaw DA, Laperriere NJ. Emergency treatment of malignant extradural spinal cord compression: an evidence-based guideline. J Clin Oncol 1998;16:1613–1624

14. Ryu SI, Chang SD, Kim DH, et al. Image-guided hypo-fractionated stereotactic radiosurgery to spinal lesions. Neurosurgery 2001;49:838–846

15. Amendola BE, Wolf AL, Coy SR, Amendola M, Bloch L. Gamma knife radiosurgery in the treatment of patients with single and multiple brain metastases from carcinoma of the breast. Cancer J 2000;6:88–92

16. Benzil DL, Saboori M, Mogilner AY, Rocchio R, Moorthy CR. Safety and efficacy of stereotactic radiosurgery for tumors of the spine. J Neurosurg 2004;101(Suppl 3):413–418

17. Bilsky MH, Yamada Y, Yenice KM, et al. Intensity-modulated stereotactic radiotherapy of paraspinal tumors: a preliminary report. Neurosurgery 2004;54:823–830

18. Chang EL, Shiu AS, Lii M-F, et al. Phase I clinical evaluation of near-simultaneous computed tomographic image-guided stereotactic body radiotherapy for spinal metastases. Int J Radiat Oncol Biol Phys 2004;59:1288–1294

19. Gagnon GJ, Henderson FC, Gehan EA, et al. Cyberknife radiosurgery for breast cancer spine metastases: a matched-pair analysis. Cancer 2007;110:1796–1802

20. Jin J-Y, Chen Q, Jin R, et al. Technical and clinical experience with spine radiosurgery: a new technology for management of localized spine metastases. Technol Cancer Res Treat 2007;6:127–133

21. Milker-Zabel S, Zabel A, Thilmann C, Schlegel W, Wannenmacher M, Debus J. Clinical results of retreatment of vertebral bone metastases by stereotactic conformal radiotherapy and intensity-modulated radiotherapy. Int J Radiat Oncol Biol Phys 2003;55:162–167

22. Ryu S, Fang Yin F, Rock J, et al. Image-guided and intensity-modulated radiosurgery for patients with spinal metastasis. Cancer 2003;97:2013–2018

23. Shiu AS, Chang EL, Ye J-S, et al. Near simultaneous computed tomography image-guided stereotactic spinal radiotherapy: an emerging paradigm for achieving true stereotaxy. Int J Radiat Oncol Biol Phys 2003;57:605–613

24. Yin FF, Ryu S, Ajlouni M, et al. Image-guided procedures for intensity-modulated spinal radiosurgery: technical note. J Neurosurg 2004;101(Suppl 3):419–424

25. Auchter RM, Lamond JP, Alexander E, et al. A multiinstitutional outcome and prognostic factor analysis of radiosurgery for resectable single brain metastasis. Int J Radiat Oncol Biol Phys 1996;35:27–35

26. Chang SD, Adler JR Jr, Hancock SL. Clinical uses of radiosurgery. Oncology (Williston Park) 1998;12:1181–1188, 1191

27. Flickinger JC, Kondziolka D, Lunsford LD, et al. A multi-institutional experience with stereotactic radiosurgery for solitary brain metastasis. Int J Radiat Oncol Biol Phys 1994;28:797–802

28. Kondziolka D, Patel A, Lunsford LD, Kassam A, Flickinger JC. Stereotactic radiosurgery plus whole brain radiotherapy versus radiotherapy alone for patients with multiple brain metastases. Int J Radiat Oncol Biol Phys 1999;45:427–434

29. Loeffler JS, Kooy HM, Wen PY, et al. The treatment of recurrent brain metastases with stereotactic radiosurgery. J Clin Oncol 1990;8:576–582

30. Sperduto P, Scott C, Andrews D. Stereotactic radiosurgery with whole brain radiation therapy improves survival in patients with brain metastases: report of radiation therapy oncology group phase III study 95–08. Int J Radiat Oncol Biol Phys 2002;54(2 Suppl 1):3

31. Hamilton AJ, Lulu BA. A prototype device for linear accelerator-based extracranial radiosurgery. Acta Neurochir Suppl (Wien) 1995;63:40–43

32. Hamilton AJ. Linear accelerator (LINAC)-based stereotactic spinal radiosurgery. In: Gildenberg PL, Tasker RR, eds. Textbook of Stereotactic and Functional Neurosurgery. New York: McGraw-Hill; 1998:857

33. Blomgren H, Lax I, Näslund I, Svanström R. Stereotactic high dose fraction radiation therapy of extracranial tumors using an accelerator: clinical experience of the first thirty-one patients. Acta Oncol 1995;34:861–870

34. Lax I, Blomgren H, Näslund I, Svanström R. Stereotactic radiotherapy of malignancies in the abdomen: methodological aspects. Acta Oncol 1994;33:677–683

35. Baisden JM, Benedict SH, Sheng K, Read PW, Larner JM. Helical TomoTherapy in the treatment of central nervous system metastasis. Neurosurg Focus 2007;22:E8

36. Chang SD, Adler JR Jr. Current status and optimal use of radiosurgery. Oncology (Williston Park) 2001;15:209–216

37. Colombo F, Pozza F, Chierego G, Casentini L, De Luca G, Francescon P. Linear accelerator radiosurgery of cerebral arteriovenous malformations: an update. Neurosurgery 1994;34:14–20

38. Gerszten PC, Burton SA, Ozhasoglu C, Welch WC. Radiosurgery for spinal metastases: clinical experience in 500 cases from a single institution. Spine (Phila Pa 1976) 2007;32:193–199

39. Gerszten PC, Welch WC. Cyberknife radiosurgery for metastatic spine tumors. Neurosurg Clin N Am 2004;15:491–501

40. Hamilton AJ, Lulu BA, Fosmire H, Stea B, Cassady JR. Preliminary clinical experience with linear accelerator-based spinal stereotactic radiosurgery. Neurosurgery 1995;36:311–319

41. Hitchcock E, Kitchen G, Dalton E, Pope B. Stereotactic LINAC radiosurgery. Br J Neurosurg 1989;3:305–312

42. Medin PM, Solberg TD, De Salles AA, et al. Investigations of a minimally invasive method for treatment of spinal malignancies with LINAC stereotactic radiation therapy: accuracy and animal studies. Int J Radiat Oncol Biol Phys 2002;52:1111–1122

43. Pirzkall A, Lohr F, Rhein B, et al. Conformal radiotherapy of challenging paraspinal tumors using a multiple arc segment technique. Int J Radiat Oncol Biol Phys 2000;48:1197–1204

44. Ryu S, Rock J, Rosenblum M, Kim JH. Patterns of failure after single-dose radiosurgery for spinal metastasis. J Neurosurg 2004;101(Suppl 3):402–405

45. Pieters RS, Niemierko A, Fullerton BC, Munzenrider JE. Cauda equina tolerance to high-dose fractionated irradiation. Int J Radiat Oncol Biol Phys 2006;64:251–257

46. Ryu S, Jin J-Y, Jin R, et al. Partial volume tolerance of the spinal cord and complications of single-dose radiosurgery. Cancer 2007;109:628–636

47. Emami B, Lyman JT, Brown A, et al. Tolerance of normal tissue to therapeutic irradiation. Int J Radiat Oncol Biol Phys 1991;21:109–122

48. Gerszten PC, Bilsky MH. Spine radiosurgery. Contemporary Neurosurgery 2006;28:1–8

49. Tong D, Gillick L, Hendrickson FR. The palliation of symptomatic osseous metastases: final results of the study by the Radiation Therapy Oncology Group. Cancer 1982;50:893–899

50. Wara WM, Phillips TL, Sheline GE, Schwade JG. Radiation tolerance of the spinal cord. Cancer 1975;35:1558–1562

51. Hatlevoll R, Høst H, Kaalhus O. Myelopathy following radiotherapy of bronchial carcinoma with large single fractions: a retrospective study. Int J Radiat Oncol Biol Phys 1983;9:41–44

52. Abbatucci JS, Delozier T, Quint R, Roussel A, Brune D. Radiation myelopathy of the cervical spinal cord: time, dose and volume factors. Int J Radiat Oncol Biol Phys 1978;4:239–248

53. McCunniff AJ, Liang MJ. Radiation tolerance of the cervical spinal cord. Int J Radiat Oncol Biol Phys 1989;16:675–678

54. Phillips TL, Buschke F. Radiation tolerance of the thoracic spinal cord. Am J Roentgenol Radium Ther Nucl Med 1969;105:659–664

55. Klish MD, Watson GA, Shrieve DC. Radiation and intensity-modulated radiotherapy for metastatic spine tumors. Neurosurg Clin N Am 2004;15:481–490

56. Rock JP, Ryu S, Yin FF. Novalis radiosurgery for metastatic spine tumors. Neurosurg Clin N Am 2004;15:503–509

57. Yamada Y, Lovelock DM, Yenice KM, et al. Multifractionated image-guided and stereotactic intensity-modulated radiotherapy of paraspinal tumors: a preliminary report. Int J Radiat Oncol Biol Phys 2005;62:53–61

58. Degen JW, Gagnon GJ, Voyadzis J-M, et al. CyberKnife stereotactic radiosurgical treatment of spinal tumors for pain control and quality of life. J Neurosurg Spine 2005;2:540–549

59. Ho AK, Fu D, Cotrutz C, et al. A study of the accuracy of Cyberknife spinal radiosurgery using skeletal structure tracking. Neurosurgery 2007;60(2, Suppl 1):ONS147–ONS156

60. Muacevic A, Staehler M, Drexler C, Wowra B, Reiser M, Tonn JC. Technical description, phantom accuracy, and clinical feasibility for fiducial-free frameless real-time image-guided spinal radiosurgery. J Neurosurg Spine 2006;5:303–312

61. Adler JR Jr, Murphy MJ, Chang SD, Hancock SL. Image-guided robotic radiosurgery. Neurosurgery 1999;44:1299–1306

62. Adler JR Jr, Chang SD, Murphy MJ, Doty J, Geis P, Hancock SL. The Cyberknife: a frameless robotic system for radiosurgery. Stereotact Funct Neurosurg 1997;69(1-4 Pt 2):124–128

63. Murphy MJ, Cox RS. The accuracy of dose localization for an image-guided frameless radiosurgery system. Med Phys 1996;23:2043–2049

64. Welsh JS, Mehta MP, Mackie TR, et al. Helical tomotherapy as a means of delivering scalp-sparing whole brain radiation therapy. Technol Cancer Res Treat 2005;4:661–662, author reply 662

65. Gerszten PC, Burton SA, Welch WC, et al. Single-fraction radiosurgery for the treatment of spinal breast metastases. Cancer 2005;104:2244–2254

66. Gerszten PC, Burton SA, Belani CP, et al. Radiosurgery for the treatment of spinal lung metastases. Cancer 2006;107:2653–2661

67. Gerszten PC, Burton SA, Quinn AE, Agarwala SS, Kirkwood JM. Radiosurgery for the treatment of spinal melanoma metastases. Stereotact Funct Neurosurg 2005;83:213–221

68. Gerszten PC, Burton SA, Ozhasoglu C, et al. Stereotactic radiosurgery for spinal metastases from renal cell carcinoma. J Neurosurg Spine 2005;3:288–295

69. Ryken TC, Meeks SL, Pennington EC, et al. Initial clinical experience with frameless stereotactic radiosurgery: analysis of accuracy and feasibility. Int J Radiat Oncol Biol Phys 2001;51:1152–1158

70. Rock JP, Ryu S, Shukairy MS, et al. Postoperative radiosurgery for malignant spinal tumors. Neurosurgery 2006;58:891–898

71. Bilsky MH, Gerszten P, Laufer I, Yamada Y. Radiation for primary spine tumors. Neurosurg Clin N Am 2008;19:119–123

72. Cohen-Gadol AA, Zikel OM, Koch CA, Scheithauer BW, Krauss WE. Spinal meningiomas in patients younger than 50 years of age: a 21-year experience. J Neurosurg 2003;98(3, Suppl):258–263

73. Conti P, Pansini G, Mouchaty H, Capuano C, Conti R. Spinal neurinomas: retrospective analysis and long-term outcome of 179 consecutively operated cases and review of the literature. Surg Neurol 2004;61:34–43

74. Dodd RL, Ryu MR, Kamnerdsupaphon P, Gibbs IC, Chang SD Jr, Adler JR Jr. CyberKnife radiosurgery for benign intradural extramedullary spinal tumors. Neurosurgery 2006;58:674–685

75. Gerszten PC, Burton SA, Ozhasoglu C, McCue KJ, Quinn AE. Radiosurgery for benign intradural spinal tumors. Neurosurgery 2008;62:887–895

76. Seppälä MT, Haltia MJ, Sankila RJ, Jääskeläinen JE, Heiskanen O. Long-term outcome after removal of spinal neurofibroma. J Neurosurg 1995;82:572–577

77. Steiner L, Leksell L, Greitz T, Forster DM, Backlund EO. Stereotaxic radiosurgery for cerebral arteriovenous malformations: report of a case. Acta Chir Scand 1972;138:459–464

78. Betti OO, Munari C, Rosler R. Stereotactic radiosurgery with the linear accelerator: treatment of arteriovenous malformations. Neurosurgery 1989;24:311–321

79. Coffey RJ, Lunsford LD, Bissonette D, Flickinger JC. Stereotactic gamma radiosurgery for intracranial vascular malformations and tumors: report of the initial North American experience in 331 patients. Stereotact Funct Neurosurg 1990;54-55:535–540

80. Colombo F, Benedetti A, Pozza F, Marchetti C, Chierego G. Linear accelerator radiosurgery of cerebral arteriovenous malformations. Neurosurgery 1989;24:833–840

81. Friedman WA, Bova FJ. Linear accelerator radiosurgery for arteriovenous malformations. J Neurosurg 1992;77:832–841

82. Steinberg GK, Fabrikant JI, Marks MP, et al. Stereotactic heavy-charged-particle Bragg-peak radiation for intracranial arteriovenous malformations. N Engl J Med 1990;323:96–101

83. Steiner L. Radiosurgery in cerebral arteriovenous malformations. In: Flamm ES J, ed. Cerebrovascular Surgery. New York: Springer-Verlag; 1985:1161–1215

84. Sinclair J, Chang SD, Gibbs IC, Adler JR Jr. Multisession CyberKnife radiosurgery for intramedullary spinal cord arteriovenous malformations. Neurosurgery 2006;58:1081–1089

85. Chang S, Hancock S, Gibbs I, et al. Spinal cord arteriovenous malformation radiosurgery. In: Gerszten PC, Ryu SI, eds. Spine Radiosurgery. New York: Thieme; 2008:123

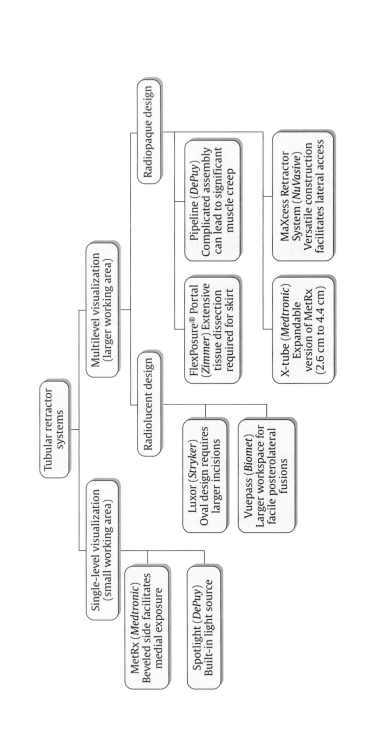

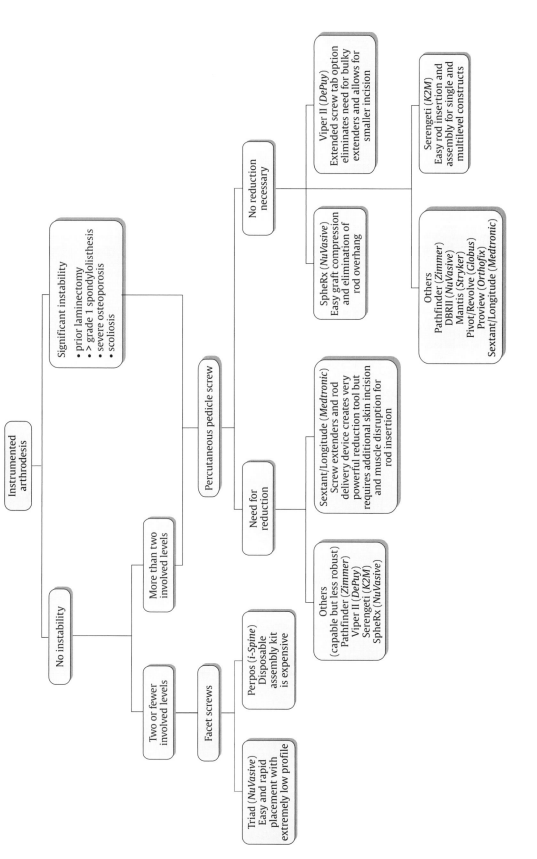

12

Minimally Invasive Instrumentation Systems

Eric K. Oerman, Zachary A. Smith, Larry T. Khoo, and Faheem A. Sandhu

Advancements in spinal surgery during the last century have been significant. Whereas complex spinal fixation was previously performed only in select centers in the early 1980s, it is now commonplace in the majority of medical centers. The growth of the field has been driven by new technologies. This includes high-quality digital fluoroscopy, which has allowed a tremendous expansion in minimally invasive spinal (MIS) techniques. MIS techniques have significant advantages because they approach the spine through a smaller corridor of dissection, leading to less iatrogenic injury and less disruption of the musculoligamentous complex.

Open procedures produce significant soft tissue injury, and it has been observed that the retractors used for posterior lumbar exposures exert significant pressure on the musculature, thereby inducing ischemia.[1] Even short procedures, such as microdiskectomy, have been shown to lead to a 30% decrease in lumbar isokinetic strength with flexion.[2] See and Kraft provided further evidence with electrophysiological studies showing chronic denervation and electromyographic (EMG) changes in the paraspinal muscles after open surgery.[3] Radiographically, this has been demonstrated by significant long-term atrophy of the operated muscle segment.[4] Sihvonen et al have directly correlated the degree of iatrogenic paraspinal injury with the increased incidence of failed back syndrome.[5] MIS techniques avoid iatrogenic injury of the posterior musculoligamentous complex. As a result, there is decreased postoperative pain, shorter hospital stays, and improved recovery times.[6–10]

This chapter summarizes some of the tools/instrumentation systems used to perform MIS procedures on the spine. There are many MIS options available to the surgeon for access and stabilization of the spine. Helping to decipher the relative advantages of the various systems is the goal of this chapter.

◆ Minimally Invasive Access/Tubular Retractor Systems

Background

The push to make surgery less invasive and to minimize damage to normal tissue structures is a common goal throughout all surgical disciplines. Starting with Yasargil's pioneering use of the operating microscope to perform a lumbar diskectomy in 1967, MIS surgery has had a renaissance in recent years due to the development of modern tubular retractor systems, which can be incorporated into almost any traditionally open procedure.[11] These retractors allow surgeons to trade the large incisions and working spaces of open surgery for small (15 to 30 mm) incisions and targeted working spaces via narrow metal channels.

In 1991, Wolfhard Caspar utilized a speculum-like retractor that can be considered a precursor to many of the current MIS tubular retractor systems to perform his variation of microsurgical diskectomy.[12] Foley and Smith introduced and popularized what can be considered the first muscle-splitting, tubular-based retraction procedure, dubbed microendoscopic diskectomy (MED), in 1997. The initial system (MED tubular retractor, Medtronic, Minneapolis, MN), was an endoscopic procedure and did not gain significant support in clinical practice due to the steep learning curve of mastering endoscopic surgery.[13] However, in 2003 the introduction of a tubular retractor system (METRx, Medtronic, Minneapolis, MN) that allowed surgeons to use the operating microscope led to popularization of tube-based procedures. Over the past decade, tubular retractors have grown in their complexity to become highly sophisticated devices incorporating expandable parts or skirts, fiberoptics, and endoscopic visualization options to aid in the performance of more complex surgical procedures.

Each of these retractors allows for a muscle-splitting approach to the spine and thus significantly less destruction of the muscular anatomy and less soft tissue retraction. Multiple investigators have demonstrated that this leads to shorter hospital stays and diminished postoperative pain.[14-16] There are several different MIS access systems available in the marketplace for surgeons to choose from. What follows is a comparative analysis of various commonly used tubular retractors (fixed and adjustable).

Select Minimally Invasive Spinal Access Systems

METRx Tubular Retractor (Medtronic)

Pros:

- Versatility—can be employed in cervical, thoracic, and lumbar procedures.
- Allows for direct visualization.
- Decreases muscle damage and tissue disruption.
- Unilateral bevel allows better medial visualization.

Cons:

- Definite learning curve in using system optimally.
- Small working area risks inadequate decompression in some cases.

- Rigid wall increases risk of cord injury when performing thoracic diskectomy unless the disk is very lateralized.

The METRx tubular retractor (Medtronic, Minneapolis, MN) is the first tubular retractor system designed to split muscles along the path of insertion, thereby reducing tissue trauma. After K-wire placement and incision, a working corridor is developed by serial dilation (**Fig. 12.1**). The great versatility of the METRx system has lent itself to use in the cervical, thoracic, and lumbar spine with predominantly posterior applications but some anterior applications as well. While the strength of the system is in facilitating MIS microdiskectomy, laminectomy, or other microscopic decompression procedures, the METRx system has been used for instrumentation

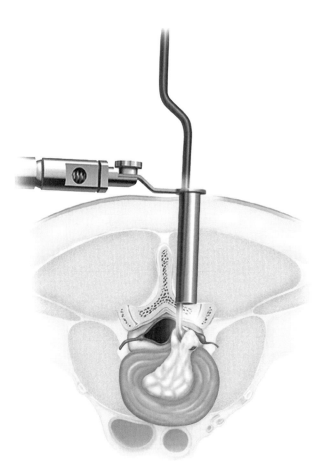

Fig. 12.1   Illustrated cross-section showing the METRx (Medtronic, Minneapolis, MN) tubular retractor passing through the paraspinal muscles and docking above the intervertebral space following successful placement. The tubular retractor is stabilized via an articulating arm affixed to the operating table. (Courtesy of Medtronic.)

with screws and rods in the cervical spine, albeit with an increased difficulty of placing rods through the small working channel.[17] The second-generation design of this retractor incorporates a bevel on one side of the working space to facilitate medial exposure. It is not recommended to use fixed-diameter tubular retractors for centralized thoracic disk herniations because the rigid wall of the tubular retractor limits the lateral angulation of instruments needed to safely work under the spinal cord to avoid injury.

Spotlight Visualization System (DePuy)

Pros:

- Built-in light source improves visualization without use of the operating microscope.
- Versatility—can be employed in cervical, thoracic, and lumbar procedures.
- Allows for direct visualization.
- Decreases muscle damage and tissue disruption.

Cons:

- Limited visualization at the base from fixed circular design.
- Definite learning curve in using system optimally.
- Small working area risks inadequate decompression in some cases.
- Rigid wall increases risk of cord injury when performing thoracic diskectomy unless the disk is very lateralized.

The Spotlight Access System (DePuy Spine, Inc., Raynham, MA) access system is a dilator-based tubular retractor very similar to the METRx system. It incorporates a built-in light source that can help eliminate shadows at the base of the working channel (**Fig. 12.2**). The fixed circular end of the working channel does limit visualization somewhat.

Vuepass (Biomet)

Pros:

- Radiolucent retractor facilitates improved fluoroscopic imaging.
- Additional cannulas can be used to expand working area.
- Expansive workspace allows for facile posterolateral fusions.

Cons:

- Standard drawbacks of other fixed tubular retractors.

The Vuepass (Biomet, Parsippany, NJ) is one of the most recently introduced MIS access technologies. The unique feature of Vuepass is that it is constructed from Makrolon, a polycarbonate thermoplastic polymer. This design choice makes it radiolucent on fluoroscopy, and makes it possible to view structures that may be obscured by the retractor while one is using fluoroscopy. In addition, Vuepass incorporates many of the features of other systems. Larger-diameter cannulas can be added to span more than one level and permit both interbody and posterolateral fusions, as

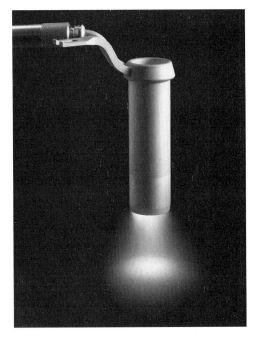

Fig. 12.2 Rendering of the integrated light source on the distal end of the Spotlight (DePuy Spine, Inc., Raynham, MA) tubular retractor. The light source can enhance direct visualization, but its utility is somewhat limited by the decreased visibility from the tube's restrictive circular geometry. (Courtesy of DePuy.)

well as other standard procedures. Its radiolucency, in addition to its other features and compatibility with any screw–rod system, make the Vuepass a versatile retraction system.

X-TUBE Dynamic Visualization System (Medtronic)

Pros:

- Versatility—can be employed in cervical, thoracic, and lumbar procedures.
- Reduced muscle damage and tissue disruption.
- Expandable base significantly increases work area compared with METRx.
- Optional integrated light source.

Cons:

- Expanded work area leads to greater tissue disruption.
- Muscle damage from overuse of monopolar coagulation.

The X-TUBE (Medtronic) is the evolution of METRx to incorporate an expandable workspace at the base of the retractor. The base can expand from 2.6 to

4.4 cm; the X-TUBE is mainly employed for performing transforaminal lumbar interbody fusion (TLIF) and posterior lumbar interbody fusion (PLIF) procedures. After K-wire placement, an incision is made and a series of tubular dilators are used to develop the working channel. Once the dilators are in place, the X-TUBE is placed over them and held in place by an articulated arm affixed to the table. Interbody fusion can be performed through the closed X-TUBE, after which the X-TUBE can be expanded to give direct visualization between adjacent pedicles in most patients. This allows for direct placement of pedicle screws and rod as well as intratransverse arthrodesis, if desired. For multilevel fusions, the X-TUBE requires multiple placements and, due to the increased operative time this can cause, for fusions exceeding three or more levels, it may be preferable to utilize an alternative approach (lateral or open).

FlexPosure® Portal Visualization System (Zimmer)

Pros:

- Expands internally to span up to two segments, thereby only requiring a small incision on each side of the spine.
- Direct visualization throughout procedure via expandable retractor with skirt.
- Allows for interbody fusion, posterolateral fusion, and direct screw and rod placement.
- Can be used for two-level fixation.

Cons:

- Less rigid wall requires extensive mobilization of tissue off the spine to optimize retraction that can lead to increased muscle damage and postoperative pain/spasm.

The FlexPosure® Portal (Zimmer, Minneapolis, MN) MIS system, sold as a complete rod and screw system as TiTLE 2® (Zimmer), is an MIS system built around a unique visualization device. Unlike other MIS systems, the FlexPosure® Portal incorporates a unique expander with a flared "skirt" at the base and a pivoting upper cannula that allows direct visualization of up to two levels of the spine (**Fig. 12.3**). This expansive range of vision permits completion of a two-level fusion performed through a small incision under direct visualization. The drawback to this method is that more extensive tissue dissection is required, thereby causing a greater perturbation of normal anatomical structures. Additionally, large multilevel fusion constructs require multiple placements of the FlexPosure® Portal retractor and therefore can take more time when compared with other approaches.

Pipeline Expandable Access System (DePuy)

Pros:

- Individually telescoping blades help prevent muscle creep.
- Curved retractor skeleton increases distal visualization while minimizing superficial exposure.

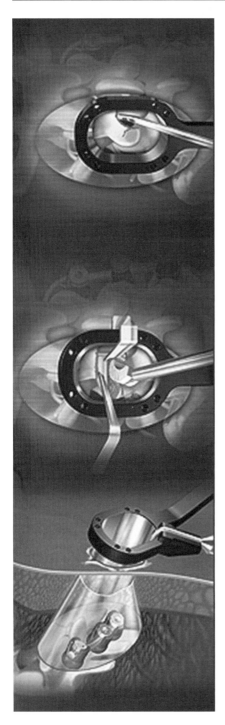

Fig. 12.3 Illustration of the FlexPosure® Portal (Zimmer, Minneapolis, MN) demonstrating its expanded viewing field and flared skirt. The lower panel demonstrates the simultaneous visualization of multiple levels via a single incision.

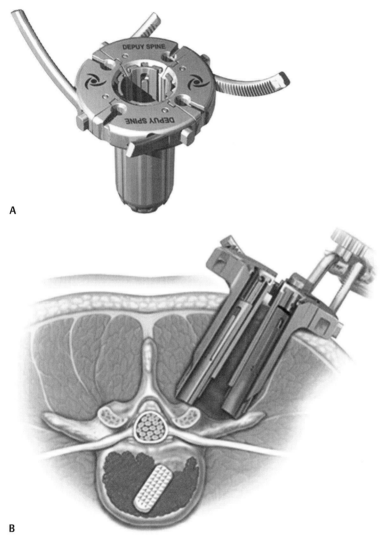

Fig. 12.4 **(A)** Illustration of the Pipeline system (DePuy Spine, Inc., Raynham, MA) showing its individually telescoping blades fully retracted. **(B)** Axial view of final medial-lateral positioning of the dilator through the multifidus and longissimus muscles. (*continued*)

- Can be expanded independently in both cephalad-caudal and medial-lateral directions to simultaneously visualize up to two levels.
- Comes in both large and small sizes and accommodates a light source.

Cons:

- Slightly complicated assembly.
- Requires larger superficial incision than other expandable retractors.

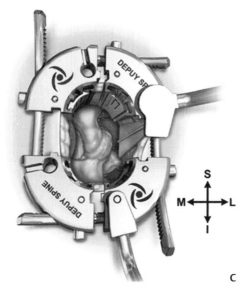

Fig. 12.4 (*continued*)   **(C)** The retractor blades are opened, providing an expansive view of an exposed facet joint. (Courtesy of DePuy.)

Pipeline (DePuy Spine, Inc., Raynham, MA) was designed primarily for posterior lumbar decompression and instrumented arthrodesis (**Fig. 12.4A–C**). Following an initial incision, the first dilator is inserted down to the lamina, and placement is confirmed via fluoroscopy prior to inserting the following three dilators. After selecting the appropriate retractor size and assembling the retractor setup, the retractor is placed over the fourth dilator using a T-handle. At this time the light source and the medial-lateral blades can be attached, in addition to affixing the retractor to the articulating arm. At any point, the telescoping blades can be advanced to help prevent tissue creep from the longissimus or multifidus muscles. Interbody fusion and direct placement of pedicle screws and rods can be achieved through the Pipeline expandable retractor.

Luxor Retractor System (Stryker)

Pros:

- Oval shape minimizes medial/lateral retraction to reduce muscle damage.
- Radiolucent retractor facilitates improved fluoroscopic imaging.
- Oval shape and cephalad-caudal expansion capabilities allow for simultaneous visualization of up to two levels.
- Light source built into retractor system for superior illumination.

Cons:

- Larger superficial incision required for maximal retraction.
- Medial and lateral exposure more limited than other retractors.

The recently introduced Luxor Minimally Invasive Retractor System (Stryker, Kalamazoo, MI) is a tubular retractor system with similar elements to both the METRx and the Vuepass. The Luxor is at heart a tubular retractor system with cephalad-caudal expansion capability, and a built-in light source that is additionally radiolucent. Beyond combining these features, the Luxor has abandoned the traditional circular shape of the tubular retractors for an oval design with its primary axis in the cephalocaudal direction in parallel with the paraspinous muscle fibers.

MaXcess Retractor System (NuVasive)

Pros:

- Can be expanded independently in both cephalocaudal and medial-lateral directions to simultaneously visualize up to two levels.
- Versatile system that can be modified as necessary with variable-length retractor blades and shim extensions making lateral access surgery very feasible.
- Light source built into retractor blades for superior illumination.
- Can be combined with Neurovision (NuVasive) for intraoperative EMG monitoring.

Cons:

- Significant muscle creep when used as a TLIF retractor.

The MaXcess retractor system (NuVasive, Inc., San Diego, CA) is a second-generation tubular retraction system that has gained significant use in performing lateral interbody fusions, although it can also be used for performing standard posterior spinal procedures. An articulating arm is attached to the retractor, which can then be adjusted in the cephalad-caudal direction by squeezing the retractor handles to expand the workspace to the desired amount. Additionally, the medial retractor blade can be adjusted independently via a knob on the side of the access driver. A fourth retractor blade is optional, and shims can be inserted down the blades to help with muscle tissue creep. Light cables can also be placed in the retractor blades for increased illumination.

Trans-sacral Access (TranS1)

Pros:

- Truly minimal access approach to L5–S1 disk, possibly L4–5, with no issues related to tissue/muscle creep.
- Good distraction capability with specially designed reverse threaded screw.

Cons:

- Limited application (L5–S1, possibly L4–5).
- No direct visualization of disk space or end plates.

The trans-sacral approach is a unique method for lower lumbar arthrodesis, and the avenue of approach affords specific advantages. Existing ventral and dorsal approaches for L5–SI arthrodesis result in damage to the annulus and disruption of either the posterior or anterior longitudinal ligament. This can contribute to biomechanical destabilization.[18] The trans-sacral approach enters the L5–SI interspace without disruption of the annulus or the surrounding ligaments. Further, the AxiaLIF (TranS1, Wilmington, NC) cage construct provides immediate and significant segmental stiffness from distraction across the disk space. The cage itself contains differential screw pitch at the ends of the cage, allowing for a wide variety of distraction heights. Lastly, the trans-sacral cage provides excellent resistance to shear, translation, and extension that surpasses that of standard interbody constructs.[19]

Initial positioning should place the patient prone on a radiolucent operative table. The anus is isolated with an occlusive dressing, and an ~15 mm incision line is prepared caudal and lateral to the paracoccygeal notch.[20] The incision is made through the skin and the underlying fascia, and blunt finger dissection is used to open the fascia. The operator then directly palpates the coccyx. The guide pin/stylet assembly is inserted into the incision and advanced along the anterior midline of the sacrum. Under fluoroscopic guidance, a guide pin introducer is engaged on the anterior cortex at the S1–2 junction. Then attention is turned toward achievement of an optimal trajectory of the stylet. In the sagittal plane, the stylet should pass through the center of the L5–S1 disk space while remaining in the anterior column of the L5 vertebral body. The guide pin is tapped, and with serial dilation an osseous working channel is developed. The final working channel is 10 mm in size. Through this working channel a 9 mm reamer can be placed for final preparation of the working space.

Diskectomy through the previously described working channel is undertaken with uniquely designed dynamic cutting-loops and disk extractors that have been designed for specific use with this application. The cutting loops are designed to be introduced in a coaxial fashion, but regain a set angle once inside the disk space. Diskectomy is followed by the use of a specifically designed brush-wire that is deployed into the disk space to capture fragmented disk material. The bone graft can now be placed into the disk space through the working channel. Finally, a large introducer cannula is inserted over the guide pin. This is used for placement of the threaded cage. The threaded cage has two unique pitches (11 mm at the L5 body with wider thread pitch and 14 mm diameter with a narrower-threaded pitch at the S1 portion). Appropriate sizing and distraction are confirmed using lateral fluoroscopic control.

Minimally Invasive Access Systems—Clinical Decision Making

Many muscle-splitting, tubular retractors are now available for surgeons to perform simple as well as complex spinal procedures. Although slight variations are present in the different systems, they all remain very similar in function. Fixed-diameter retractors can be readily used for performing diskectomies, decompressions, and even interbody fusions, whereas expandable retractors also allow for placement of spinal instrumentation and multilevel surgery. Not mentioned in this discussion are several retractors designed to allow surgeons to perform "mini-open" procedures as a bridge between standard open surgery and tubular-based retractor surgery. These include Quadrant (Medtronic), AccuVision (Biomet), MARS (Globus Medical, Inc., Audubon, PA), and Terra Nova (K2M, Inc., Leesburg, VA).

The decision as to which system to use is somewhat arbitrary because most allow for adequate completion of the desired surgical procedure. Surgeon familiarity, either through residency/fellowship training or company-sponsored training courses, is the most common basis for deciding on the system to use for a minimal access procedure. Once a surgeon is facile with performing MIS procedures, direct comparison of different systems can be done to aid in deciphering relative advantages between systems.

◆ Minimally Invasive Posterior Thoracolumbar Instrumentation

Background

Failure of stand-alone interbody arthrodesis led many surgeons to supplement fusion constructs with posterior pedicle screw and rod instrumentation.[21,22] This practice of supplementing fusion constructs with thoracolumbar hardware is supported by biomechanical studies. They demonstrate that early segmental fixation enhances the stiffness of the fusion construct with axial-compressive, axial-torque, and flexion-extension loads.[23-25] The first attempt at MIS instrumentation was Magerl's percutaneous insertion of pedicle screws with external fixation for spinal instability in 1980.[26] Further initial surgical experience with MIS segmental fusion involved pedicle screws connected to subcutaneous plates placed above the dorsal fascia.[14,26] These early attempts at MIS fusion were complicated by the superficial (and suprafascial) location of the construct. Hardware removal was often necessary because of both patient discomfort and nonunion.[14,15,26]

One of the initial MIS systems with widespread use was the Sextant system (Medtronic Sofamor Danek, Memphis, TN). Designed by Foley and colleagues in 2001, the system allowed for pedicle cannulation using a vertebroplasty-type approach. Following placement of the screws, the rod is passed into place using a geometrically constrained pathway that triangulates the two screw heads and the rod tip.[15] The limitations of this system are primarily related to the arc-type rod insertion. This has specific relevance for cases with hyperlordotic curves, severe deformity, and multi-level fusions. In addition, the system does not have a portal for direct visualization of the screw heads or rod path.

Some of the limitations inherent with Sextant are overcome by the Pathfinder® system (Zimmer, Minneapolis, MN), a more recent addition to the growing suite of MIS thoracolumbar fusion systems. This system utilizes a "letter-opener" technique to develop a soft tissue plane between pedicles. Extender sleeves allow direct connection to the screw, and the rod is guided down each sleeve vertically into the working plane. An even more revolutionary system is the recently introduced Serengeti (K2M, Inc., Leesburg, VA) system for percutaneous stabilization. The Serengeti utilizes disposable screw-based sleeves for soft tissue retraction allowing direct visualization of screw heads during rod placement. Additionally, the screw sleeves can serve as the basis for building a retractor that allows for the rapid assembly of a multilevel fusion construct with minimal tissue disruption. NuVasive has also recently introduced a similar screw-based retractor system dubbed the MAS. These screw-based retractors represent the latest evolution in minimal access to the spine for arthrodesis procedures. All of these systems use a muscle-splitting approach to the pedicle and thus significantly less distortion of the muscular and ligamentous anatomy and less soft tissue retraction. Multiple investigators have demonstrated that this results in shorter hospital stays and diminished postoperative pain.[14-16]

Select Thoracolumbar MIS Rod and Screw Systems

Sextant/Longitude MIS Rod and Screw System (Medtronic Sofamor Danek)

Pros:

- Strong reduction capability.
- Geometrical constraints allow for facile rod insertion.
- Can be used for multilevel fixation.

Cons:

- Requires an extra incision and muscle dissection for rod placement.
- Arc-rod insertion can be difficult with large deformities or lordotic changes.
- Screw insertion at L5–S1 can be challenging due to proximity of screw extenders.

Placement of pedicle screws with the use of the Sextant system can be done with either conventional fluoroscopy, alternated between anteroposterior (AP), lateral, and oblique trajectories, or with use of neuronavigation. Initially, the Jamshidi needle is advanced through the pedicle into the vertebral body. Needle placement is guided primarily in the oblique view using the pedicle markings determined during setup. The needle location is confirmed within the posterior portion of the centrum, and the central obturator of the needle is removed. A K-wire is then exchanged through the working channel of the needle. This technique is repeated at the adjacent pedicle(s). The first of three METRx tissue dilators is inserted over the K-wire to dilate the fascia, and the inner two dilators are removed. Following a preparatory tap, cannulated screws are attached to screw extenders and inserted over the K-wire. Each Sextant pedicle screw is made of titanium and is multiaxial, with excellent profile and fatigue resistance. The screws vary in length from 35 to 55 mm. The screw extenders are then coupled and the Sextant device is attached to the screw assembly. A stab incision is then made and a tissue path is created with the trochar. A rod is then attached to the inserter and passed through the screw heads, followed by set caps.

Design characteristics unique to Sextant include the screw extenders and the geometric arch that is designed for rod placement (**Fig. 12.5**). The extender units have an opening in the saddle for the rod. It places the screw saddles in alignment so they can be connected to the rod after placement. Additionally, the percutaneous pathway and arc are designed to bisect the screw heads. Each rod is precontoured in a curvilinear fashion to match the contour of insertion and normal lumbar lordosis. Ultimately this design allows for facile rod placement and has a strong reduction capability due to the Sextant inserter being connected to the extender units and rod following insertion and prior to fixation.

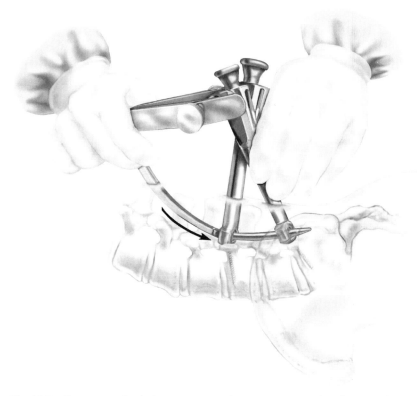

Fig. 12.5 Illustration of rod placement using the Sextant system (Medtronic Sofamor Danek, Memphis, TN). The geometric constraints of the unique arc–rod device allow for facile placement by constraining the pathway that the rod can traverse. (Courtesy Medtronic Sofamor Danek.)

Pathfinder® MIS Rod and Screw System (Zimmer)

Pros:

- Minimizes retraction to better maintain anatomical stability.
- Can be used for multilevel fixation.

Cons:

- Can encounter difficulties due to no direct visualization of rod insertion.

The Pathfinder® (Zimmer) MIS pedicle screw system is a more recent system for MIS thoracolumbar instrumentation. Similar to other MIS systems, the Pathfinder® system is a top-loading unit with cannulated polyaxial screws. The system provides screws of 5.5 , 6.5, and 7.5 mm and contains pre-bent rods designed specifically to match extender sleeves. Screw fixation is undertaken using a standard approach

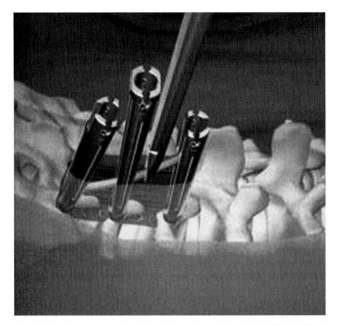

Fig. 12.6   Demonstration of rod insertion with the Pathfinder® system (Zimmer, Minneapolis, MN). The pre-bent rod is inserted into specifically matched extender sleeves attached to each of the polyaxial screw heads. (Courtesy Zimmer, Minneapolis, MN.)

of pedicle cannulation with a Jamshidi needle and then followed by sequential dilation with four muscle dilators. The final dilator serves as a 19 mm access port. The extender sleeves in this system allow for a direct connection with the screw. Unique to this system is the development of the soft tissue plane between pedicles with a "letter opener" technique. This uses a metallic tissue dilation wedge that is moved longitudinally in the working plane to develop a path for the rod. The rod is guided down the extender sleeve vertically and progressively aligns itself to a horizontal orientation as it enters the working plane and engages the tulip heads (**Fig. 12.6**).

Viper II MIS Rod and Screw System (DePuy)

Pros:

- Extended tab screws eliminate need for extenders and require smaller (15 mm) incisions for insertion.
- Can be used for multilevel fixation.

Cons:

- Can encounter difficulties due to no direct visualization of rod insertion.

The Viper II (DePuy) MIS pedicle screw system is a more recent system for MIS thoracolumbar instrumentation. Designed to minimize soft tissue trauma and difficulty of rod insertion, the Viper II, in addition to standard screw extenders, employs a unique extended tab screw (X-Tab) system that eliminates the need for extenders and necessitates smaller (15 mm) incisions that allow for rapid screw placement and rod reduction. Additionally, the Viper II is versatile enough to be employed from the thoracic region to the sacrum using either precontoured rods or on-site contoured rods from 30 mm to 480 mm long, as the situation demands. An additional feature worth mentioning in the context of the Viper II's versatility is its compatibility with the Expendium (Depuy) vertebral body derotation set for scoliosis correction. Rod insertion is done in a top-loading manner from one end of the construct and does not require an additional skin incision or significant tissue disruption. Like other systems without direct visualization of rod insertion, however, the placement of the Viper II's rods must be done via indirect markers and tactile feedback, thereby predisposing the system to potential rod insertion difficulties.

SpheRx/DBR II Rod and Screw System (NuVasive)

Pros:

- No rod overhang minimizes potential for construct causing adjacent-level symptoms.
- Easy graft compression upon cap tightening.
- Integrates with NeuroVision intraoperative EMG system.
- Can be used for multilevel fixation.

Cons:

- Can encounter difficulties due to no direct visualization of rod insertion.
- Difficult to control rod orientation on final placement due to the design of the rod inserter.

SpheRx/DBR II (NuVasive) cannulated pedicle screws are a recent addition to the suite of thoracolumbar MIS systems. Like other percutaneous systems, the SpheRx lacks direct visualization of rod insertion and can therefore incur further soft tissue damage due to extra manipulation of the rod during insertion. This problem is slightly compounded in the SpheRx due to the design of the rod inserter, which can make control of the rod's orientation on final placement difficult. Despite these insertion drawbacks, the rods of the SpheRx themselves offer several distinct advantages. Their precut design and seamless integration with the screw heads create a system with no rod overhang, thereby decreasing the risk of adjacent-level degeneration. Another useful feature is that the guides themselves can be used to provide up to 5 mm of reduction via manual manipulation. Also, like the NuVasive retractors, specialized pedicle access needles can integrate with the NeuroVision EMG for intraoperative nerve root monitoring.

Serengeti Rod and Screw System (K2M)

Pros:

- Screw-based retractors provide a fixed window that allows for direct visualization of screw placement and eliminate retractor repositioning.

- Retractable sleeves make for easy rod insertion, even with multilevel fixation.
- No interference of screw extenders for fixation at L5 and S1.
- Can be used for multilevel fixation.
- Smallest inner cannulation of percutaneous pedicle screws increases screw strength.

Cons:

- Difficulty with sleeve breakage or removal if screws are inserted to flush with the facet.
- Head orientation of the screws can be lateralized on rod insertion making set cap application difficult.
- Care is required to avoid bending less rigid guide wires.

The Serengeti (K2M) MIS pedicle screw system is a recent system for MIS thoracolumbar instrumentation that is optimized for multilevel instrumentation. Similar to other MIS systems, the Serengeti system is a top-loading unit with cannulated polyaxial screws. Serengeti's primary innovation is placing the screws into flexible plastic retractor sleeves, which allows for retractor and screw placement in a single step. Repeating this process at multiple levels allows for a facile and rapid construction of a multilevel fusion construct (**Fig. 12.7**). Additionally, rod insertion, even for

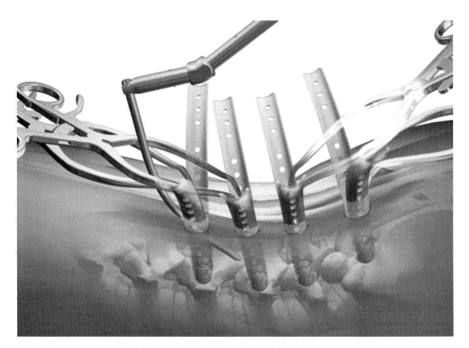

Fig. 12.7 Illustration of rod placement into the flexible plastic retractor sleeves of the Serengeti system (K2M, Inc., Leesburg, VA). The rod is being inserted through one of the end screw retractor sleeves to rapidly create a multilevel fusion construct. (©2010 K2M. All rights reserved. Used with the permission of K2M.)

long constructs, can be done through one of the end screw retractor sleeves. Cap assembly and compression can then be done under direct visualization.

Select Thoracolumbar MIS Facet Screw Systems

Triad Facet Screw System (NuVasive)

Pros:

- Percutaneous placement of full-thread or lag screws allows for rapid placement.
- Easier to place than pedicle screws and requires less tissue dissection.
- Very low hardware profile.
- Can be used for multilevel fixation.
- Can be readily placed in the lateral position.

Cons:

- Cautioned use in the presence of severe degenerative disease of the facet joint.
- Inherently less rigid system.
- May not provide sufficient support for large multilevel fusions utilizing anterior cages.

The Triad (NuVasive) is a percutaneous facet screw system. One midline incision is made through which the double-threaded lag screws can be placed over a K-wire. This procedure can rapidly be replicated bilaterally and at multiple levels for facile stabilization, though it is accepted that more rigid pedicle screw–rod systems may be more appropriate for larger fusion constructs or in cases of instability.

PERPOS Facet Screw System (Interventional Spine)

Pros:

- Easier to place than pedicle screws and requires less tissue dissection.
- Allows for compression of the facet joint.
- Very low hardware profile.
- Can be used for multilevel fixation.
- Can be placed in the lateral position.

Cons:

- Cautioned use in the presence of severe degenerative disease of the facet joint.
- Inherently less rigid system.
- May not provide sufficient support for large multilevel fusions utilizing anterior cages.
- Significant cost due to disposable kit assembly.
- Single size may not be ideal for all clinical scenarios.

The PERPOS facet screw system (Interventional Spine, Inc., Irvine, CA) is one of the first percutaneous facet screw systems and was designed to combine the advantages of minimally invasive percutaneous placement with the advantages of facet compression upon fixation. A single midline skin incision is made through which the double-threaded lag screws can be placed over a K-wire. This procedure can rapidly be replicated bilaterally and at multiple levels for rapid multilevel stabilization. The uniqueness of this system is the capability of compression of the facet joint upon placement of the facet screw.

Thoracolumbar MIS—Clinical Decision Making

Judicious use of MIS techniques requires an understanding of the drawbacks and advantages of these procedures. The learning curve that must be overcome before a surgeon is technically proficient is not insignificant, particularly in the case of percutaneous procedures where direct anatomical visualization is minimized. In almost all of the procedures, standard landmarks are often not fully exposed, which can further disorient the surgeon. In addition, MIS is technically demanding due to working in a small area and with longer (bayoneted) instruments. Therefore, when deciding to use MIS techniques surgeons must first determine their level of comfort. However, the use of MIS has many advantages. The development of a working channel between muscle planes permits access with the potential for less muscular disruption, leading to less pain and shorter hospital stays. In our experience, blood loss is markedly decreased, and patients have smaller incisions and better healing. A balance between these competing drawbacks and advantages should be the initial step in decision making.

◆ Conclusion

The development of MIS systems is a reflection of the progressive refinement of widely accepted operative techniques. Frequently, the techniques used in MIS work through the same corridors of entry as have been used traditionally. In other MIS techniques, like eXtreme Lateral Interbody Fusion (XLIF, NuVasive) or AxiaLIF (TranS1), the technique uses a novel means of access. Yet, regardless of the corridor of access, each of these procedures is a direct extension of traditional spinal techniques. The same goals are achieved as with open surgery, and with similar efficacy.

The use of minimally invasive access continues to have tremendous growth. This has been driven by both surgeons as well as patients. Although the initial experience in the field was with simple decompression techniques, MIS has developed applications for PLIF, TLIF, thoracolumbar posterolateral fusion, posterior cervical fixation, and anterior lumbar interbody arthrodesis. Expansion into new corridors of access, as evidenced by trans-sacral fusion and screw-based retractors, provides further development of the field. As clinical medicine continues to demand shorter hospital stays and quicker recovery, the development of new techniques in MIS procedures will provide a new framework for development and innovation. This will determine the means by which we provide future care for spinal disease and improved patient outcomes.

References

1. Styf JR, Willén J. The effects of external compression by three different retractors on pressure in the erector spine muscles during and after posterior lumbar spine surgery in humans. Spine (Phila Pa 1976) 1998;23:354–358

2. Kahanovitz N, Viola K, Gallagher M. Long-term strength assessment of postoperative diskectomy patients. Spine (Phila Pa 1976) 1989;14:402–403

3. See DH, Kraft GH. Electromyography in paraspinal muscles following surgery for root compression. Arch Phys Med Rehabil 1975;56:80–83

4. Mayer TG, Vanharanta H, Gatchel RJ, et al. Comparison of CT scan muscle measurements and isokinetic trunk strength in postoperative patients. Spine (Phila Pa 1976) 1989;14:33–36

5. Sihvonen T, Herno A, Paljarva L, Airaksinen O, Partanen J, Tapaninaho A. Local denervation atrophy of paraspinal muscles in postoperative failed back syndrome. Spine 1993;18:575–581

6. Fessler RG, Khoo LT. Minimally invasive cervical microendoscopic foraminotomy: an initial clinical experience. Neurosurgery 2002;51(5, Suppl):S37–S45

7. Ratliff JK, Cooper PR. Cervical laminoplasty: a critical review. J Neurosurg 2003;98(3, Suppl):230–238

8. Hosono N, Yonenobu K, Ono K. Neck and shoulder pain after laminoplasty: a noticeable complication. Spine (Phila Pa 1976) 1996;21:1969–1973

9. Aldrich F. Posterolateral microdisectomy for cervical monoradiculopathy caused by posterolateral soft cervical disc sequestration. J Neurosurg 1990;72:370–377

10. Foley KT, Holly LT, Schwender JD. Minimally invasive lumbar fusion. Spine (Phila Pa 1976) 2003;28(15, Suppl):S26–S35

11. Yasargil MG. Microsurgical operation of herniated lumbar disc. In: Wullenweber R, Brock M, Hamer J, Klinger M, Spoerri O. Advances in Neurosurgery. Vol 4. Berlin: Springer-Verlag; 1977:81–94

12. Faubert C, Caspar W. Lumbar percutaneous discectomy: initial experience in 28 cases. Neuroradiology 1991;33:407–410

13. Oppenheimer JH, DeCastro I, McDonnell DE. Minimally invasive spine technology and minimally invasive spine surgery: a historical review. Neurosurg Focus 2009;27:E9

14. Lowery GL, Kulkarni SS. Posterior percutaneous spine instrumentation. Eur Spine J 2000;9(Suppl 1):S126–S130

15. Foley KT, Gupta SK, Justis JR, Sherman MC. Percutaneous pedicle screw fixation of the lumbar spine. Neurosurg Focus 2001;10:E10

16. Khoo LT, Palmer S, Laich DT, Fessler RG. Minimally invasive percutaneous posterior lumbar interbody fusion. Neurosurgery 2002;51(5, Suppl):S166–S171

17. Wang MY, Prusmack CJ, Green BA, Gruen JP, Levi AD. Minimally invasive lateral mass screws in the treatment of cervical facet dislocations: technical note. Neurosurgery 2003;52:444–447

18. Marotta N, Cosar M, Pimenta L, Khoo LT. A novel minimally invasive presacral approach and instrumentation technique for anterior L5–S1 intervertebral discectomy and fusion: technical description and case presentations. Neurosurg Focus 2006;20(1):E9

19. Slosar PJ, Reynolds JB, Koestler M. The axial cage. A pilot study for interbody fusion in a higher-grade spondylolisthesis. Spine 2001;1:115–120

20. Trambert JJ. Percutaneous interventions in the presacral space: CT guided precoccygeal approach—early experience. Radiology 1999;213:901–904

21. Steffee AD. The variable screw placement systems with posterior lumbar interbody fusion. In: Lin PM, Gill K, eds. Lumbar Interbody Fusion: Principles and Techniques of Spine Surgery. Rockville, MD: Aspen Publishers; 1989:81–95

22. Wiltse LL. Surgery for intervertebral disk disease of the lumbar spine. Clin Orthop Relat Res 1977;129:22–45

23. Boult M, Fraser RD, Jones N, et al. Posterior Lumbar Interbody Fusion. 2nd ed. New York: Raven Press; 1993

24. Brodke DS, Dick JC, Kunz DN, McCabe R, Zdeblick TA. Posterior lumbar interbody fusion: a biomechanical comparison, including a new threaded cage. Spine (Phila Pa 1976) 1997;22:26–31

25. Lin PM, Cautilli RA, Joyce MF. Posterior lumbar interbody fusion. Clin Orthop Relat Res 1983;180:154–168

26. Magerl F. Verletzungen der Brust- und Lendenwirbelsaule. Langenbecks Arch Chir 1980; 352:428–433

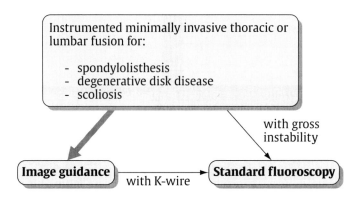

13

Image Guidance in Minimally Invasive Spine Surgery

Eric A. Potts

Image guidance is at the heart of all spine surgery. Conventional means of image guidance, in the form of radiography or fluoroscopy, are used during nearly every spine procedure. The evolution of image guidance has paralleled the evolution of surgical techniques for the treatment of spine pathology. This evolution has led to the introduction of modern image guidance systems, which employ intraoperatively acquired, multiplanar images to navigate manipulation of spinal elements and placement of hardware in real time via a computer workstation. Image-guided spinal surgery has become safer and more efficient with further advancement of its associated technology. A description of this technology will be the focus of this chapter.

The role of image guidance to enhance the safety and efficacy of complex spine surgery is well documented.[1–8] This technology can improve the accuracy and efficiency of the techniques used for decompression of the neural elements and placement of instrumentation, therefore ensuring effective stabilization while protecting the neighboring neurovascular elements. In addition, this method dramatically reduces or eliminates the surgeon's exposure to radiation.[9] Despite the aforementioned advantages, this technology has been, unfortunately, poorly and slowly adopted by all spine surgeons.

◆ The Evolution of Image-Guided Spine Surgery

Image-guided spine surgery has evolved to its current form through a step-by-step improvement in three-dimensional (3-D) imaging technology, which can be applied in the operating room environment to localize spinal bony elements accurately and reliably. Initially, in the 1990s, the use of two-dimensional (2-D) spine surgery imaging to guide surgery was onerous and mastered by few surgeons. The process had several limitations: first, a preoperative computed tomographic (CT) scan was required and then imported to a computer workstation in the operating room. After a reference array was affixed to the patient, the surgeon chose a series of anatomical landmarks on the workstation and co-registered the corresponding landmarks on the patient to the ones preselected on the workstation.[1] Unlike the relative ease of touching preplaced fiducials on the head for cranial neuronavigation, arriving at the preselected point in the spine was difficult. If an acceptable error range was not met, then a surface merge was employed. This process entailed co-registering 50 to 100 points on the spine. Finally, the surgeon was ready to navigate the *one* level attached to the reference array; navigating away from the frame decreased the accuracy. Re-registering multiple levels was usually a time-prohibitive exercise. Whereas navigating "open" posterior procedures was cumbersome, navigating minimal access or anterior procedures was impossible. Once the hardware was placed, conventional means, including postoperative imaging, were employed to verify proper hardware placement.

Although most neurosurgeons easily adopted the technology for their cranial cases, few employed it for the spine. The barriers to success for image guidance in spine surgery can be grouped into the following:

1. A need for additional preoperative imaging
2. A relatively extended intraoperative time commitment requiring
   a. Point to point registration and providing
   b. A limited range of navigation
3. Availability of only 2-D versus 3-D images
4. Reliance on old technology for verification of placement of instrumentation, including
   a. Conventional radiographs and fluoroscopy
   b. Pedicle screw stimulation
   c. Postoperative imaging requiring return of the patient to the operating room if hardware position is not satisfactory
5. Cost constraints

The next foray was virtual fluoroscopy.[10] In this circumstance, a standard C-arm was fitted with a calibration target, and multiple 2-D images were obtained and transferred to a computer workstation intraoperatively. There was no need to register anatomical points or employ surface merging because the images were only in 2-D. Although the system allowed multiple images to be displayed, real-time biplanar views were available with*out* a need for a C-arm. Nevertheless, the accuracy and effectiveness of this technology were questioned in some studies.[11] Given that the patient was imaged in the operative position using this imaging technique, navigating around multiple segments may have been associated with less error. Virtual fluoroscopy overcame two of the barriers to the adoption of image guidance in spine surgery: the need for preoperative imaging, and extended intraoperative time commitment. However, this technique also suffered from shortcomings: providing only 2-D images and requiring postoperative imaging for confirmation of instrumentation position.[10] Some surgeons believed this technique did not add enough value to warrant its routine use in everyday practice. Although this method eliminated radiation exposure to the surgeon, it eventually failed to gain widespread popularity.

In 2002, Siemens introduced the Iso-C 3-D image guidance system.[12] This technology was revolutionary and served as a foundation that led to the development of today's image guidance systems. Iso-C is a motorized C-arm that acquires and reformats multiple 2-D images into a 3-D dataset and provides multiplanar images intraoperatively.[13] This development obviated the need for a preoperative scan and the imaging of the patient in a position different from the operative position.[14] Most importantly, intraoperative 3-D imaging became a reality.

For the first time, intraoperative 3-D confirmation of instrumentation position was available before leaving the operating room.[14] Unfortunately, some shortcomings remained evident: the image quality was not always acceptable, especially for obese patients,[13,14] and for images at the cervicothoracic junction, the initial scans had a limited field of view (typically three lumbar vertebrae), and scanning took ~2 minutes.

Moreover, the presence of prior instrumentation significantly degraded the image quality. Although this was a quantum leap in advancing image guidance for spine surgery, it also faced a limited acceptance. The advocates of the old-style 3-D systems touted its better image quality, whereas others failed to see a clear benefit for immediate feedback and the opportunity for intraoperative 3-D confirmation of instrumentation position.

In 2006, Breakaway Imaging (Littleton, MA), funded in part by spine surgeons, released the O-arm. This modality has the same functionality as Iso-C but provides a vastly improved image quality and field of view. The O-arm can image up to four or five lumbar segments, six thoracic segments, or the entire cervical spine, and it provides good-quality images despite the presence of prior instrumentation and obesity. The O-arm is able to adequately image the previously considered "difficult to image areas" such as the cervicothoracic junction. In fact, scans may be done with the retractors in place. Additionally, a scan takes less than 25 seconds to complete. This device lifted most of the barriers to the widespread adoption of image guidance during spine surgery. One limitation of this modality is its inability to guide K-wires; the presence of a K-wire demands real-time imaging with fluoroscopy. The only other remaining barrier has been the cost of the device. In the current health care economy, it may be impossible for all spine surgeons, especially in small medical centers, to have access to cutting-edge navigation technology. The O-arm itself costs in excess of $600,000. A more cost-effective option that can provide navigation to a larger subset of surgeons is greatly needed.

As the advantages of more minimal-access procedures are recognized and used by surgeons, the normal anatomical landmarks become less visible intraoperatively, and the importance of image guidance is more evident. Intraoperative image guidance can increase the accuracy and efficiency of instrumentation placement and ensure adequacy of neural decompression or diskectomy. Furthermore, this method can significantly decrease the extent of radiation exposure to the surgeon. These superior qualities allow for the introduction of further innovative applications for image guidance in the future.

◆ Application of Image Guidance to Minimally Invasive Spine Surgery

During minimal-access posterior lumbar fusion procedures, including posterior lumbar interbody and transforaminal lumbar interbody fusions (PLIFs and TLIFs), safe screw implantation can be effectively navigated. Typically, the reference arc is attached to the iliac crest (**Fig. 13.1**) or a neighboring spinous process. Following

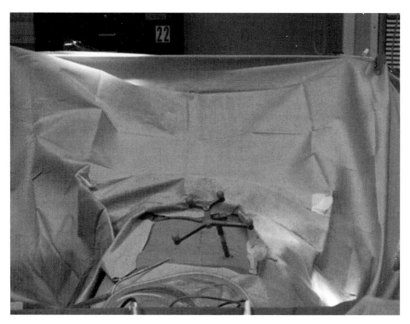

Fig. 13.1 The percutaneous reference arc attached to the posterior ilium. This allows access to the surgical site seen above the arc.

the completion of an initial scan, real-time navigation and proper positioning of the incisions are possible. Care must be taken to avoid displacement of the reference arc. To eliminate the need for multiple scans, pedicles are accessed initially, prior to completing the diskectomy. If this order is reversed, the application of the intervertebral spacer will most likely displace the neighboring pedicles and introduce inaccuracy in navigation. Instrumentation can be placed in the contralateral pedicles (**Fig. 13.2**). On the ipsilateral side, depending on the instrumentation system used, the prepared bony tracts for the hardware can be left empty, or K-wires can be used as placeholders.

Initially, cannulated pedicle screws and K-wires were used for instrumentation. An image-guided Jamshidi needle was used to develop the pedicle tract. The most effective method was to impact the needle with a mallet. By using image guidance and the O-arm we are able to visualize the exact trajectory of the Jamshidi needle and ensure proper positioning. Trajectory views provide a sagittal-type and axial-type orthogonal view to the Jamshidi needle (**Fig. 13.2**). These views supplement the typical anteroposterior (AP) and lateral views that are obtained with conventional fluoroscopy. Once the pedicle and vertebral body are accessed, a K-wire is left in the anterior third of the vertebral body. Taps and screws can be delivered over the K-wires with periodic fluoroscopic shots to ensure the K-wire is not migrating.

We have now moved to a method that does not need guide wires for placement of pedicle screws. This obviates the need for live fluoroscopy. An awl–tap combination is used in conjunction with a tissue protector and the navigation system. Our workflow now begins with a navigable dilator to mark the incision and trajectory. A tissue

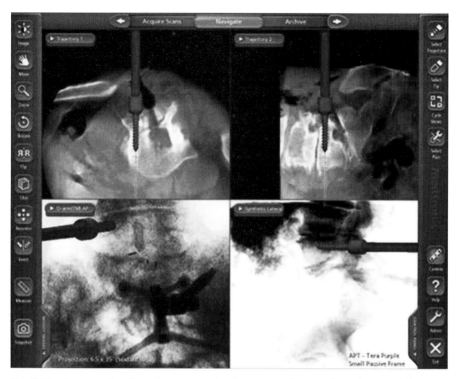

Fig. 13.2   A screen shot from the neuronavigation system showing the right L5 pedicle screw being placed with a neuronavigation-compatible screwdriver. This allows for real-time tracking of the screw position within the vertebral body. Also visible in the upper right frame is the percutaneous reference arc within the ilium.

protector is passed over the dilator and the dilator is removed. The navigable awl–tap is introduced down the tissue protector. Screw length and size are determined by a projection while the awl–tap is resting on the starting point for the pedicle screw. A surgical plan for the screw is saved on the computer workstation. The awl–tap is then advanced through the pedicle into the vertebral body. The awl–tap and tissue protector are removed together and the pedicle screw is then delivered using a navigable screw driver. The previously saved surgical plan allows the surgeon to find the correct starting point and correct trajectory.

Image guidance can be employed for facetectomy, contralateral decompression, and diskectomy (**Fig. 13.3**). Verifying an adequate neural decompression is often helpful, especially during contralateral diskectomy. After placement of a TLIF or PLIF spacer, ipsilateral screws can be implanted. Prior to leaving the operating room, a confirmatory scan can be obtained to ensure good hardware position and allow for a chance to reposition the hardware, if necessary. This greatly decreases or possibly eliminates a second surgery for malpositioned screws.

The instrumentation system used should be integrated with the navigation system. Although intraoperative navigation is a powerful tool, K-wire-based instrumentation

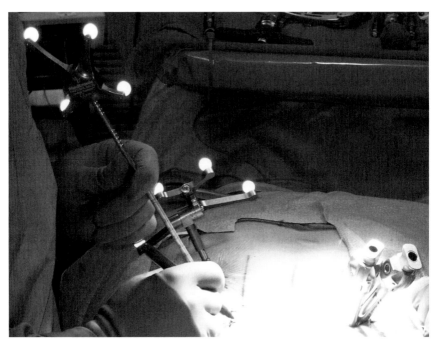

Fig. 13.3 Contralateral pedicle screw extenders are seen on the right side of the image. A navigable probe is being used to plan the 1 in. incision for facetectomy and interbody arthrodesis. A percutaneous reference arc is also seen in this image.

systems require live fluoroscopy for wire insertion to monitor for the inadvertent advancement of the wires in undesirable routes.

This same technique can be used during posterior thoracic instrumentation. If interbody spacers are not used, then instrumentation can be placed anytime during the procedure. A common concern has remained the accuracy of image guidance while navigating away from the reference arc. This concern was evaluated in a study by Lekovic et al, who found no decrease in the accuracy over the entire length of the thoracic spine with one fixed reference arc positioned at either the top or the bottom part of the construct.[15] Papadopoulos et al also found similar findings in the lumbar spine.[16]

As the application of minimal access techniques is expanded, image guidance will find a further role in spine surgery. Currently, posterior thoracic and lumbar corpectomies are being attempted with increasing frequency. The anatomy of the region in these procedures is often challenging and neighbored by important neurovascular structures that require further technology, such as image guidance to monitor and assist with surgical manipulation around the "hard-to-see" corners. Image guidance can confirm the adequacy of decompression and assist with proper implant positioning. Finally, image guidance can be used to localize operative levels in any minimal access lumbar procedure.

A common misconception is that image guidance adds a significant amount of time to the operative procedure. Nottmeier and Crosby have recently shown that multiple levels can be scanned in an efficient manner with an average time of less than 9 minutes with little or no radiation exposure to the surgeon or staff.[17] Sasso and Garrido[18] have also shown that image guidance for lumbosacral fusion may, in fact, decrease operative time.

◆ Potential Pitfalls of Image-Guided Surgery

Navigation can be particularly useful during complex procedures or revision cases where normal anatomy may not be readily visualized. The strategy to reserve navigation for only these cases is flawed and can lead to poor adoption of the technique by the surgeon and the operating room staff. Navigation changes the workflow of the operating room during surgery. This change impacts not only the surgeon but also the radiation technologist, the circulating nurse, and the scrub technician. Frequent use of this technology will improve the navigation experience for all the involved personnel, whereas exclusive use in difficult cases will only introduce yet another unfamiliar variable.

Most modern image-guided systems use infrared cameras (**Fig. 13.4**). This leads to one of the common changes required in the workflow of the operating room. Any object blocking the line of sight between the camera and the navigated instrument and the reference arc will render navigation ineffective. The next challenge is to leave the reference arc undisturbed. The longer the operative time and the more manipulation present around the arc, the more likely the arc position may change, rendering navigation inaccurate. We, therefore, recommend the use of navigation as soon as the reference images are available.

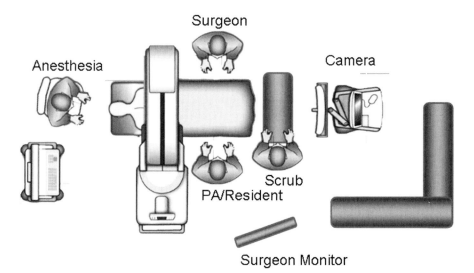

Fig. 13.4   A typical operating room setup is shown here. The camera is positioned at the foot of the bed for the majority of thoracolumbar procedures. Surgeon monitor is placed across the table for easy viewing. In integrated operating rooms, more than one surgeon monitor is employed for easy viewing from both sides of the table.

Although modern image guidance is highly accurate, a complete "blind" reliance on navigation is not advisable. This blind faith in the technology can be alluring, but it must be remembered that navigation is not a substitute for sound clinical judgment. Navigation is best thought of as a powerful adjunct to capable surgical skills.

Reference Arc Options

The reference arc must be attached to a nonmobile area. A common option for attachment is a spinous process for "open" cases, or the pelvis (posterior ilium) for minimal-access cases. However, for navigation in the cervical and upper thoracic spine, the pelvis is not desirable due to its distance from the area to be navigated and instrumented. In these cases, a spinous process may remain a good option to anchor the reference arc. In addition, during the surgical treatment of patients with a profound spinal instability, repeat imaging while placing the reference arc in different levels may be necessary to ensure acceptable accuracy.

Radiation Exposure

The radiation dose to the surgeon and operating room staff during minimally invasive procedures is not well documented. Recently, Bindal et al reported radiation exposure in a small series of minimally invasive TLIFs.[19] The mean dose to the collar, waist, and hand of the operating surgeon was 32, 27, and 76 mRem, respectively. Using these numbers, the surgeon would exceed the allowed annual dose to the torso after 194 cases. In a cadaveric study of radiation exposure, Rampersaud et al found the radiation exposure for spinal procedures is in the range of 10 to 12 times the dose involved in other musculoskeletal procedures.[20]

The National Council on Radiation Protection and Measurements recommends a maximum whole-body dose of 5 Rem per year.[19,20] The International Commission on Radiologic Protection and Measurements has revised their limits to 2 Rem per year. The ALARA (as low as reasonably achievable) concept continues to hold true. There is no safe dose of radiation. These recommended limits are *maximum* doses and all efforts should be aimed at minimizing the exposure. The personnel who are exposed to greater than 10% of these limits are to be regularly monitored.[20] Unfortunately, a cavalier attitude toward radiation exposure is present among spine surgeons, and few surgeons routinely wear radiation badges. In the preceding two studies, both surgeons were very skilled in the placement of instrumentation and cognizant of the hazards of ionizing radiation. The dose to the less skilled or less careful surgeon is truly unknown.

When K-wires are not used, image guidance can *eliminate* radiation exposure to the surgeon. During image acquisition, the entire operating room team can be shielded behind lead screen or can stand outside the room. An additional benefit to the surgeon is the improved ergonomics with the elimination of the C-arm and lead aprons.

Adoption

Conversion from fluoroscopy to image guidance is challenging. As with any new procedure there is a learning curve that surgeons will experience. Image guidance can be employed in all cases. The only exception may be cases with overt instability. The quickest adoption of this technology comes with its use in all posterior thoracolumbar

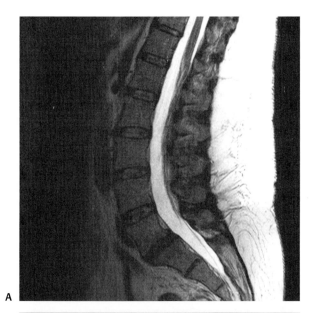

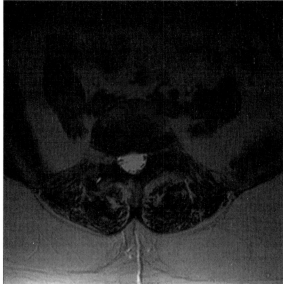

Fig. 13.5 **(A)** Preoperative T2 sagittal magnetic resonance imaging (MRI) showing grade I spondylolisthesis of L5–S1. **(B)** Preoperative T2 axial MRI through the L5–S1 level demonstrating a foraminal disk protrusion on the left. (*continued*)

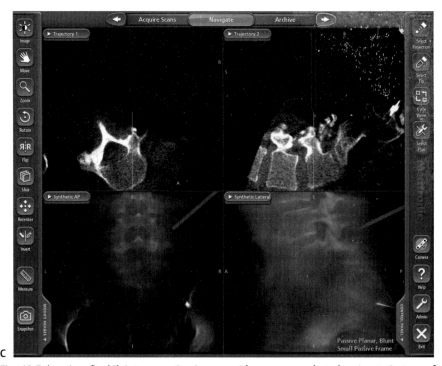

C

Fig. 13.5 (*continued*) **(C)** Intraoperative image guidance screen shot showing trajectory of the right L5 pedicle screw. Upper images are cross-sectional images obtained with the O-arm (Breakaway Imaging, Littleton, MA). Lower images are conventional fluoro shots from the O-arm. The thin line coming off the probe in the upper panels notes trajectory. Please note that by convention in the image guidance system the right side of the anatomy appears on the right side of the screen.

cases. Just as the conversion from printed films to PACS systems caused trepidation due to the rapidity of its implementation, changing all cases to image guidance seems a radical plan. But in most cases PACS has been accepted as superior to printed film, just as a familiarity with image guidance will show its clear advantages over fluoroscopy.

◆ Conclusion

Image-guided technology has greatly improved the safety and efficacy of minimal-access and complex spine surgery. The use of higher-generation image guidance systems is associated with a learning curve and requires a certain level of discipline from the operating room staff. Attention to the details mentioned in the present chapter will enable the surgeon to maximize the potential of image guidance systems in spine surgery.

Case History and Illustration

A 50-year-old woman presents with refractory left lower extremity pain, low back pain, and a mild left foot drop (**Fig. 13.5A–E**).

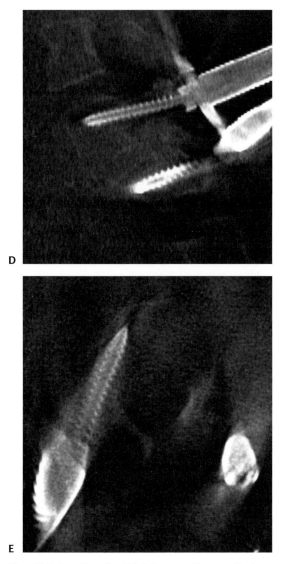

D

E

Fig. 13.5 (*continued*) **(D)** Intraoperative postinstrumentation O-arm scan. This sagittal reformat shows the trajectory of the right L5 pedicle screw. This trajectory mirrors that which was seen on the image guidance. Please note the Sextant screw extenders are still in place, allowing for adjustment of rod position or screw trajectory. **(E)** Intraoperative postinstrumentation O-arm scan. This axial reformat shows the trajectory of the right L5 pedicle screw. This trajectory mirrors that which was seen on the image guidance. Please note the Sextant screw extenders are still in place, allowing for adjustment of rod position or screw trajectory.

References

1. Holly LT, Foley KT. Intraoperative spinal navigation. Spine (Phila Pa 1976) 2003;28(15, Suppl): S54–S61

2. Kotani Y, Abumi K, Ito M, et al. Accuracy analysis of pedicle screw placement in posterior scoliosis surgery: comparison between conventional fluoroscopic and computer-assisted technique. Spine (Phila Pa 1976) 2007;32:1543–1550

3. Lim MR, Girardi FP, Yoon SC, Huang RC, Cammisa FP Jr. Accuracy of computerized frameless stereotactic image-guided pedicle screw placement into previously fused lumbar spines. Spine (Phila Pa 1976) 2005;30:1793–1798

4. Metz LN, Burch S. Computer-assisted surgical planning and image-guided surgical navigation in refractory adult scoliosis surgery: case report and review of the literature. Spine (Phila Pa 1976) 2008; 33:E287–E292

5. Nottmeier EW, Seemer W, Young PM. Placement of thoracolumbar pedicle screws using three-dimensional image guidance: experience in a large patient cohort. J Neurosurg Spine 2009;10:33–39

6. Rajasekaran S, Kamath V, Shetty AP. Intraoperative Iso-C three-dimensional navigation in excision of spinal osteoid osteomas. Spine (Phila Pa 1976) 2008;33:E25–E29

7. Rajasekaran S, Vidyadhara S, Ramesh P, Shetty AP. Randomized clinical study to compare the accuracy of navigated and non-navigated thoracic pedicle screws in deformity correction surgeries. Spine (Phila Pa 1976) 2007;32:E56–E64

8. Youkilis AS, Quint DJ, McGillicuddy JE, Papadopoulos SM. Stereotactic navigation for placement of pedicle screws in the thoracic spine. Neurosurgery 2001;48:771–778

9. Gebhard FT, Kraus MD, Schneider E, Liener UC, Kinzl L, Arand M. Does computer-assisted spine surgery reduce intraoperative radiation doses? Spine (Phila Pa 1976) 2006;31:2024–2027

10. Foley KT, Simon DA, Rampersaud YR. Virtual fluoroscopy: computer-assisted fluoroscopic navigation. Spine (Phila Pa 1976) 2001;26:347–351

11. Mirza SK, Wiggins GC, Kuntz CT IV, et al. Accuracy of thoracic vertebral body screw placement using standard fluoroscopy, fluoroscopic image guidance, and computed tomographic image guidance: a cadaver study. Spine (Phila Pa 1976) 2003;28:402–413

12. Newly available, newly approved: new products, indications, and services. Am J Orthop 2001;30:530

13. Hott JS, Papadopoulos SM, Theodore N, Dickman CA, Sonntag VK. Intraoperative Iso-C C-arm navigation in cervical spinal surgery: review of the first 52 cases. Spine (Phila Pa 1976) 2004;29:2856–2860

14. Holly LT, Foley KT. Three-dimensional fluoroscopy-guided percutaneous thoracolumbar pedicle screw placement. Technical note. J Neurosurg 2003;99(3, Suppl):324–329

15. Lekovic GP, Potts EA, Karahalios DG, Hall G. A comparison of two techniques in image-guided thoracic pedicle screw placement: a retrospective study of 37 patients and 277 pedicle screws. J Neurosurg Spine 2007;7:393–398

16. Papadopoulos EC, Girardi FP, Sama A, Sandhu HS, Cammisa FP Jr. Accuracy of single-time, multilevel registration in image-guided spinal surgery. Spine J 2005;5:263–267

17. Nottmeier EW, Crosby T. Timing of vertebral registration in three-dimensional, fluoroscopy-based, image-guided spinal surgery. J Spinal Disord Tech 2009;22:358–360

18. Sasso RC, Garrido BJ. Computer-assisted spinal navigation versus serial radiography and operative time for posterior spinal fusion at L5-S1. J Spinal Disord Tech 2007;20:118–122

19. Bindal RK, Glaze S, Ognoskie M, Tunner V, Malone R, Ghosh S. Surgeon and patient radiation exposure in minimally invasive transforaminal lumbar interbody fusion. J Neurosurg Spine 2008;9:570–573

20. Rampersaud YR, Foley KT, Shen AC, Williams S, Solomito M. Radiation exposure to the spine surgeon during fluoroscopically assisted pedicle screw insertion. Spine (Phila Pa 1976) 2000;25:2637–2645

14

Promising Advances in Minimally Invasive Spine Surgery

Richard G. Fessler

"Prescience" is not so much the ability to see the future as it is the ability to see where the future must go. It is in this sense of the word that I have pursued my career, and also in which I write this chapter. In which direction minimally invasive spine surgery (MISS) will progress is impossible to know, especially in the context of the current uncertainties of health care in America. As explained by the eminent athlete and philosopher, Yogi Berra: "It's hard to make predictions, especially about the future."

Nonetheless, having defined prescience as I have above, I am obviously going to argue that MISS *must* progress and become the mainstream technique of performing spinal surgery. On what basis would I make such a strong statement? Simply put, there is no doubt in my mind that, in skilled hands, MISS is better for patients. Ample literature now exists demonstrating that spinal surgery performed through MISS technique results in less pain and less use of pain medicine,[1,2] less blood loss,[3] lower infection rates,[4] less requirement for intensive care,[5] and less hospitalization.[3] Physiological stress is reduced.[6] Complication rates in high-risk patients are reduced.[7] Fusion rates are higher.[8] Muscle atrophy is reduced,[9] and normal motion is more accurately preserved.[10] I see no reason why nearly all spinal surgery could not be performed via MISS.

That being said, for MISS to continue to grow, advancements in several areas are necessary. These fall into the defined areas of instrumentation, image guidance, and education. Among these, the most challenging for the surgeon is education, for advanced MISS requires a significantly higher technical skill level than open surgery, and a much greater three-dimensional understanding of anatomy.

◆ Instrumentation

Although basic instrumentation has come a long way since our early attempts at MISS, available "tools" still have significant limitations. Take for example the most common MISS procedure performed, minimally invasive lumbar diskectomy. Many systems are available to perform this surgery, but all have limitations. If we first consider the area of visualization, limitations exist whether the technology is endoscopic or microscopic. On the one hand, endoscopic visualization gives one the advantage of excellent image quality of the working area and the tip of the instrument without the instrument's handle and the surgeon's hand obstructing the operative field, and without the "hassle" of bumping the instruments into the microscope lens when entering or exiting the wound. The price paid for this advantage, however, is the necessity of working in a two-dimensional visual field with a moderately bulky camera lens obstructing part of the working channel.

To circumvent the frustration many surgeons expressed in attempting to perform endoscopic minimally invasive diskectomies, tubular retractors and instruments were designed to enable surgeons to use the same technologies using microscopic visualization. This solved the problem of working in a two-dimensional visual field, but, as already indicated, created the problems of having the surgeon's hands and shaft of the instrument in the relatively narrow visual field, thus obstructing a clear view of the surgical site. To partially address this problem, bayoneted instruments were developed. These did help remove the surgeon's hands, but not the instrument's shaft, from the visual field. Furthermore, in many instances, making an instrument bayoneted impairs the function of that instrument. For example, because the working mechanism of a straight curette is achieved through turning the cutting edge at the tip of the instrument, bayoneting the shaft fundamentally changes the motion necessary to turn the tip and significantly impairs the effectiveness of the instrument. As the complexity of the surgical procedure increases, the limitations imposed by the instrumentation is compounded.

Given the limitations to endoscopic technique, are there other reasons why one might wish to utilize endoscopic rather than microscopic surgical technique? Yes. Several surgeries have significant ergonomic advantages when one is utilizing MISS technique. For example, MISS cervical foraminotomy/diskectomy can be performed with the patient either sitting or prone. To reach the operative site when using the microscope with the patient in the sitting position, the surgeon's arms must extend the entire length of the microscope for the duration of the surgery. A more comfortable position, of course is to do the microscopic foraminotomy with the patient in the prone position. However, the epidural venous plexuses surrounding the cervical nerve roots are abundant and can lead to profuse bleeding. In the patient in the prone position, this bleeding rapidly collects in the limited space of the tubular retractor and obscures the lens, making visualization difficult to impossible. However, using the endoscope with the patient in the sitting position both alleviates the discomfort of prolonged extension of the arms and the problem of excessive bleeding. Therefore, endoscopic cervical foraminotomy is one of the procedures where the endoscope has significant advantages over the microscope. Similar ergonomic advantages exist for microendoscopic vs microscopic decompression of lumbar stenosis.

Therefore, one of the directions in which MISS must move is to make "endoscopic" MISS more acceptable to surgeons. This will require the development of a user-friendly, three-dimensional camera that can fit into the confines of a relatively small tubular retractor while leaving enough room for the surgeon to work comfortably. Furthermore, it must be adaptable to multiple types of retractors, zoom, and focus.

What about more complex procedures, such as vertebrectomies, correction of scoliosis, and intradural pathology? As the complexity of the procedure increases, so does the technical demand on the surgeon and on the instrumentation. Unfortunately, despite the increased level of procedural complexity, the availability of appropriate instruments and devices proportionally decreases. What has become abundantly apparent, however, is that the larger the "open" surgical procedure, the greater the benefit to the patient if it can be done through MISS. Therefore, there is clear reason to pursue the more complicated procedures through MISS. To perform these more complicated procedures, therefore, instrumentation needs to be modified specifically for these procedures. For example, retractors now are adequate, but not great. Although they work well in the lumbar spine, where the musculature is predominantly parallel to the spine, they do not work well in the more complicated anatomical environment of the posterior cervical spine. For vertebrectomies, drills need to be slimmed down and modified to extend slightly longer. Furthermore, protective sleeves need to be readily available for each drill bit head design, to protect the surrounding structures in limited visual fields. Microinstruments need to be designed to be used through tubes and yield the same delicacy as when used under a microscope. Instruments need to be designed to easily close the dura. Finally, in major reconstructive cases, such as correction of scoliosis, de-rotation instruments, compression and distraction devices, and in situ bending instruments need to be developed.

◆ Image Guidance

One of the keys to really advancing minimally invasive surgery, and making it available to all surgeons, is the availability of affordable, user-friendly, and reliable image guidance. Three-dimensional knowledge of the spine and its surrounding soft tissue structures is critical to safely performing MISS. However, the transfer of two-dimensional fluoroscopic imaging to three-dimensional anatomy is not easy for all surgeons. Current technology has come a long way toward helping in that regard with intraoperative computed tomographic (CT) imaging. Reliability has increased significantly but is still limited by its dependence on the fixation, and lack of movement, of the reference frame during the entire time image guidance is used. Other areas in which improvements will help the surgeons are (1) improved and more widely available "guidable" instruments that accurately reflect the typical working instruments needed to complete the surgical procedure, (2) image technology that does not rely on "line of sight" imaging between the camera and imaging array, (3) less bulky equipment (the O-arm, Breakaway Imaging, Littleton, MA, for example, is huge), and (4) more time-efficient technology.

Among the major concerns of individuals considering adopting a minimally invasive technique for spinal surgery is their increased exposure to radiation. CT-based image guidance may significantly decrease this and thus make these techniques more acceptable to surgeons. Although no significant differences were found during specific surgical subsections of the transforaminal lumbar interbody fusion (TLIF) procedure, Kim et al recently reported that "total" exposure to radiation time was decreased from 147 seconds to 57 seconds using navigation-assisted fluoroscopy vs standard fluoroscopy.[11] Similarly, using CT-based image guidance, Gebhard et al reported a decrease from 177 seconds to 75 seconds of total radiation time.[12] If, as already discussed, ease and reliability of use can be improved over time, this decreased exposure to radiation will likely shift the imaging technique toward CT-based image guidance.

◆ Education

Finally, education is perhaps the key component to moving MISS into the mainstream of spinal surgery. It is generally true that new technologies take one to two generations to become widely adopted. That is certainly true of MISS. This is partly a result of what must be learned, but it is also influenced by the nature of graduate and postgraduate education.

For example, in the case of endoscopic MISS, learning the technique is particularly challenging due to the multiple skills that must be simultaneously mastered. First, the techniques (basic and "pearls") of an entirely new set of instruments and retractors must be learned. As any surgeon knows, although new instruments can be successfully used rather quickly, becoming truly facile with them takes some time. Second, learning the visual and proprioceptive skills to operate in a two-dimensional visual field can be challenging. Third, learning to work through a restrictive "tube," which requires using instruments parallel to each other, rather than triangulating, can be difficult. This is increased by the fact that instruments often collide with each other (i.e., "fight") in areas out of the visual field, making it difficult to understand why the tips of the instruments aren't doing what is intended for them. Add to these difficulties the challenge of learning how to achieve hemostasis in this environment, and the frustration level can become high. Finally, since maneuverability is restricted in the smaller tubes, performing tasks such as closing the dura can become quite difficult. When all of these are taken together, it is easy to understand the reluctance of many experienced surgeons to replace their routine and successful operations with MISS technique.

The adoption of MISS technique will also be impacted by the nature of graduate and postgraduate education. Surgical residents who are being trained in institutions in which MISS is already being widely used will simply learn this as part of their armamentarium. As more and more institutions have skilled faculty, this will become standard of care, similar to the way in which spinal instrumentation was adopted in the United States over the last 25 to 30 years. Given this rate of adoption, it is likely that spinal surgeons approaching the end of their active career will never need to learn these techniques. However, that leaves a large group of surgeons who were not trained in MISS during residency but who have long careers ahead of them and will need to learn the techniques to continue to perform surgery. Because this is not the type of surgery that can be adequately learned in a weekend course, the question is, How do these surgeons learn these techniques?

Current recommendations to acquire this training include a series of educational steps. First, one or more didactic courses should be attended to learn the indications, contraindications, and theory and basic techniques for MISS procedures. Second, hands-on training should be completed, both on foam bone models and on cadavers. Third, the student-surgeon should observe several procedures being performed by an experienced MISS surgeon. Finally, if the opportunity exists, it would also be reasonable for the less experienced MISS surgeon to "scrub" on several cases for proctoring prior to independently engaging in the procedures. It is the latter suggestion that is particularly problematic for surgeons because few centers are available where this is actually possible.

◆ Cost versus Efficacy

The advance toward MISS, of course, raises additional questions that will need to be addressed. In discussing the need for improved instrumentation and image guidance technologies, one has to wonder if the additional cost is justified. In particular, the cost of CT guidance is exorbitant. New retractor and surgical instrumentation also adds to the cost of these procedures, as does the use of new biologic agents to augment fusion, such as bone morphogenetic protein (BMP). These costs may partially or totally be offset by shorter hospital stays, decreased medical resource utilization, higher fusion rates, lower complication rates, and faster return to work, but little reliable data on these questions is available at this time. To become "mainstream," MISS must have equal or superior results compared with open surgery. Moreover, it cannot be too much more expensive. As these procedures become more frequently utilized over the next few years, the cost and comparative efficacy will be more stringently analyzed. Those procedures that are equally or more effective than their open-surgery counterparts and are equal or lower in cost will replace open surgery as the procedure of choice. Those that do not meet those criteria will fall out of use.

◆ Summary

In summary, the short-term advantages of minimally invasive spine surgery are abundantly apparent at this point. Data are slowly accumulating that the long-term benefit is significant as well. It seems, therefore, that MISS will become a common, if not the most common, technique for performing routine spine surgery. To reach that point, however, limitations on instrumentation, imaging, and training must be overcome. Moreover, strict evaluation of the clinical and cost-effectiveness of these procedures will profoundly impact their adoption.

References

1. Fessler RG, Khoo LT. Minimally invasive cervical microendoscopic foraminotomy: an initial clinical experience. Neurosurgery 2002;51(5, Suppl):S37–S45
2. O'Toole JE, Sheikh H, Eichholz KM, Fessler RG, Perez-Cruet MJ. Endoscopic posterior cervical foraminotomy and discectomy. Neurosurg Clin N Am 2006;17:411–422

3. Khoo LT, Palmer S, Laich DT, Fessler RG. Minimally invasive percutaneous posterior lumbar interbody fusion. Neurosurgery 2002;51(5, Suppl):S166–S181

4. O'Toole JE, Eichholz KM, Fessler RG. Surgical site infection rates after minimally invasive spinal surgery. J Neurosurg Spine 2009;11:471–476

5. Eichholz KM, O'Toole JE, Fessler RG. Thoracic microendoscopic discectomy. Neurosurg Clin N Am 2006;17:441–446

6. Huang TJ, Hsu RW, Li YY, Cheng CC. Less systemic cytokine response in patients following microendoscopic versus open lumbar discectomy. J Orthop Res 2005;23:406–411

7. Rosen DS, O'Toole JE, Eichholz KM, et al. Minimally invasive lumbar spinal decompression in the elderly: outcomes of 50 patients aged 75 years and older. Neurosurgery 2007;60:503–509

8. Christie SD, Kiberd MB, Song JK, Abraham E, Hrubes M, Fessler RG. Open vs MAST lumbar interbody fusion. Journal of Minimally Invasive Surgery, Submitted

9. Bresnahan L, Fessler RG, Natarajan RN. Evaluation of change in muscle activity as a result of posterior lumbar spine surgery using a dynamic modeling. Spine 2010;35(1b):E761–767

10. Bresnahan L, Ogden AT, Natarajan RN, Fessler RG. A biomechanical evaluation of graded posterior element removal for treatment of lumbar stenosis: comparison of a minimally invasive approach with two standard laminectomy techniques. Spine (Phila Pa 1976) 2009;34:17–23

11. Kim CW, Lee YP, Taylor W, Oygar A, Kim WK. Use of navigation-assisted fluoroscopy to decrease radiation exposure during minimally invasive spine surgery. Spine J 2008;8:584–590

12. Gebhard FT, Kraus MD, Schneider E, Liener UC, Kinzl L, Arand M. Does computer-assisted spine surgery reduce intraoperative radiation doses? Spine (Phila Pa 1976) 2006;31:2024–2027

Index

Note: Page numbers followed by *f* and *t* indicate figures and tables, respectively. Narratives for cineangiography are indicated by page numbers followed by *ca*.

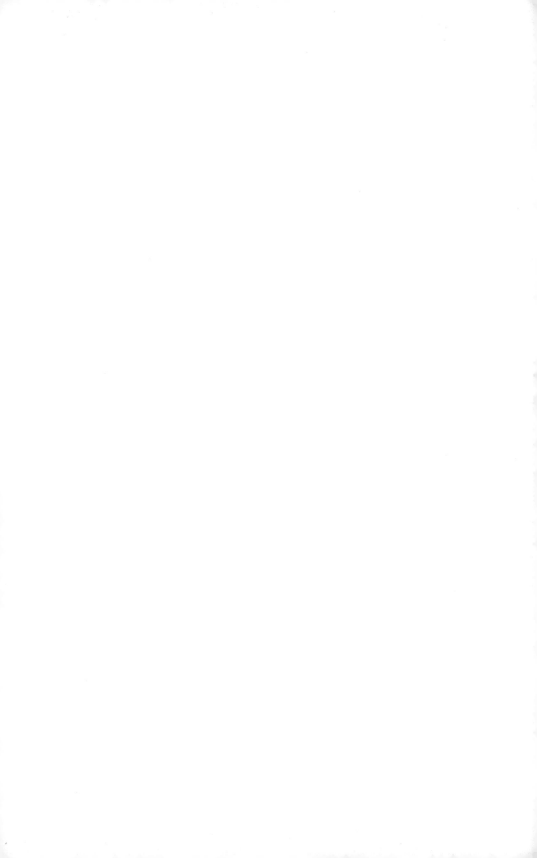